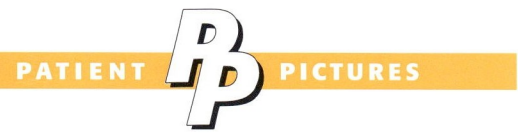

PATIENT PICTURES

Clinical drawings for your patients

Erectile dysfunction

by Christine M Evans MB ChB MD FRCS FRCS Ed
Consultant Urologist, Glan Clwyd Hospital, Rhyl, UK
and
Philip Kell MB BS MRCOG MFFP Dip GUM (LSA)
Consultant Physician, The Archway Sexual Health Clinic,
Whittington Hospital, London, UK

Series Editor: J Richard Smith MD MRCOG
Consultant Gynaecologist,
Chelsea and Westminster Hospital, London,
and Honorary Senior Lecturer in Obstetrics and Gynaecology,
Imperial College School of Medicine, London, UK

Illustrated by Dee McLean, MeDee Art, London, UK

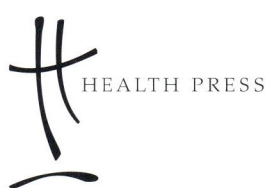

HEALTH PRESS

Oxford

Patient Pictures – Erectile dysfunction
First published 2000

Text © 2000 Christine M Evans, Philip Kell
© 2000 in this edition Health Press Limited
Health Press Limited, Elizabeth House, Queen Street,
Abingdon, Oxford OX14 3JR, UK
Tel: (01235) 523233
Fax: (01235) 523238

Patient Pictures is a trade mark of Health Press Limited.

The publisher and authors have made every effort to ensure
the accuracy of this book, but cannot accept responsibility
for any errors or omissions.

A CIP catalogue record for this title is available from the
British Library.

ISBN 1-899541-11-X

Printed by Fine Print (Services) Ltd, Oxford, UK.

Reproduction authorization

The purchaser of this *Patient Pictures* series title is hereby authorized to reproduce by photocopy only, any part of the pictorial and textual material contained in this work for non-profit, educational or patient education use. Photocopying for these purposes only is welcomed and free from further permission requirements from the publisher and free from any fee.

The reproduction of any material from this publication outside the guidelines above is strictly prohibited without the permission in writing of the publisher and is subject to minimum charges laid down by the Publishers Licensing Society Limited or its nominees.

Sarah Redston

Publisher, Health Press Limited, Oxford

Authors' preface

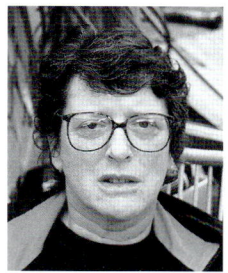

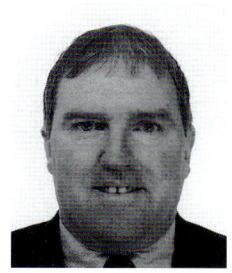

Although impotence, or erectile dysfunction (ED), has been known about for many years, until the early 1980s, the only available treatments were a pat on the back, hormone replacement, yohimbine and semi-rigid prostheses. Intrapenile, or intracorporeal, injections then became the mainstay of treatment. Although many men couldn't accept or tolerate the injections, diabetic men on insulin found the treatment both acceptable and easily learned. A proportion of patients recovered spontaneously from their ED. Still, many men were too shy or scared to seek treatment. Counselling, hormone replacement and penile prostheses all improved, and intraurethral medication was developed. In the past 2 years, however, there has been an explosion in interest, and ED is no longer the taboo subject it once was. At last, a reasonably safe, very effective oral treatment for ED exists. This, at present, needs to be prescribed by medical practitioners, though we only have the word of our patients that they have a problem with their erections.

ED is an important medical problem that causes untold distress both to men and their partners. The aim of this book is to let patients know that something can be done and to help them understand the choices.

Christine M Evans MB ChB MD FRCS FRCS Ed
Consultant Urologist, Glan Clwyd Hospital, Rhyl, UK
and
Philip Kell MB BS MRCOG MFFP Dip GUM (LSA)
Consultant Physician, The Archway Sexual Health Clinic,
Whittington Hospital, London, UK

The penis

- The penis is the male organ that contains the urethra, the channel through which urine and semen leave the body.

- The penis consists of the base (closest to the body), the shaft and the glans (furthest from the body).

- The penis is attached at the base to the bony pelvis.

- The shaft, the main body of the penis, consists of three columns of erectile tissue. It has two side parts (the corpora cavernosa) and a central part (the corpus spongiosum). The central part is close to the surface and surrounds the urethra. The corpora cavernosa are cylinders of spongy tissue, each surrounded by fibrous tissue (the tunica albuginea). They have a honeycomb-like structure that contains muscle and fills with blood following sexual stimulation to produce an erection.

- The glans is the acorn-shaped region at the tip of the penis. It is an extension of the corpus spongiosum. The meatus or urethral opening, at the end of the urethra, is in the glans. In an uncircumcised man, the glans is covered by the foreskin.

Cross-section of the shaft of the penis

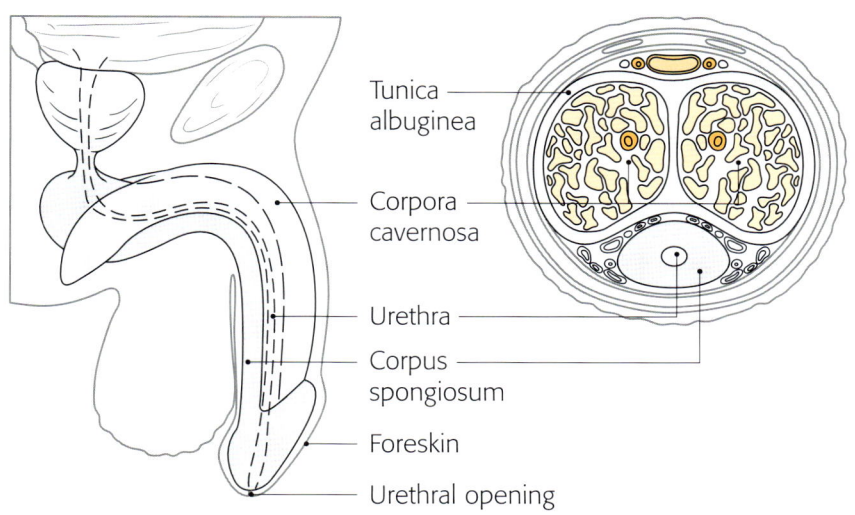

Tunica albuginea

Corpora cavernosa

Urethra

Corpus spongiosum

Foreskin

Urethral opening

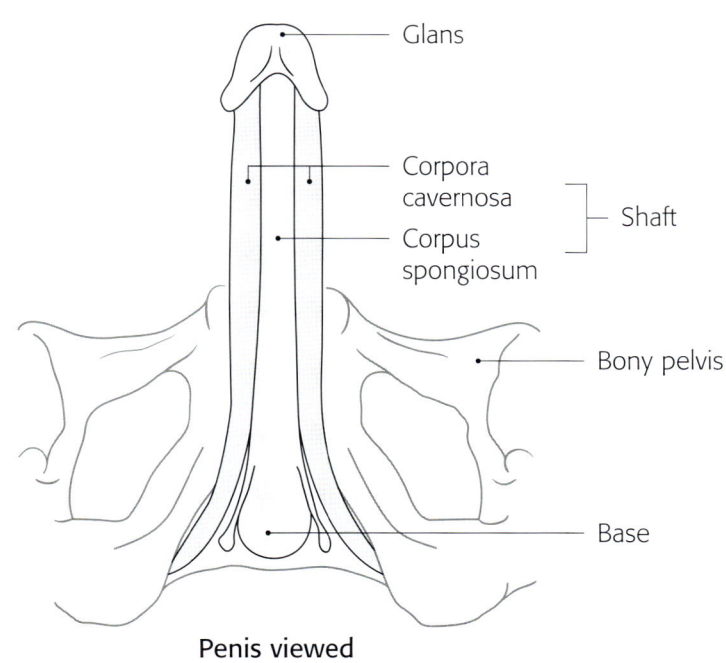

Glans

Corpora cavernosa

Corpus spongiosum

Shaft

Bony pelvis

Base

Penis viewed from beneath

Physical changes during an erection

- When the penis is limp or flaccid, it is under the control of the sympathetic nervous system, which is responsible for reflex, or unconscious, actions. The blood vessels are narrow and the blood flow is low, keeping the penis small.

- Sexual stimulation occurs when you see or hear things that arouse you, or you are touched sexually. The part of the nervous system that has an opposite effect from the sympathetic nervous system (the parasympathetic nervous system) becomes active, making the blood vessels wider and the cavernosal tissue of the penis fill with blood.

- The increased blood in the penis compresses the veins against the fibrous tissue (the tunica albuginea) around the corpora. Because of the increased pressure, less blood leaves the penis. An erection occurs.

- After ejaculation (when semen is discharged from the penis), the penis becomes limp. This is called detumescence. The sympathetic nervous system takes over again.

Limp

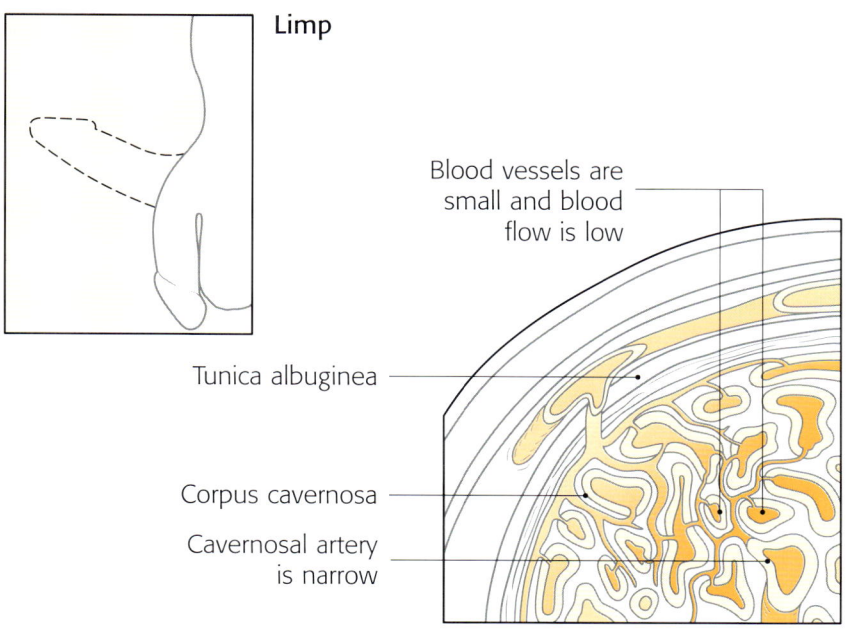

Blood vessels are small and blood flow is low

Tunica albuginea

Corpus cavernosa

Cavernosal artery is narrow

Erect

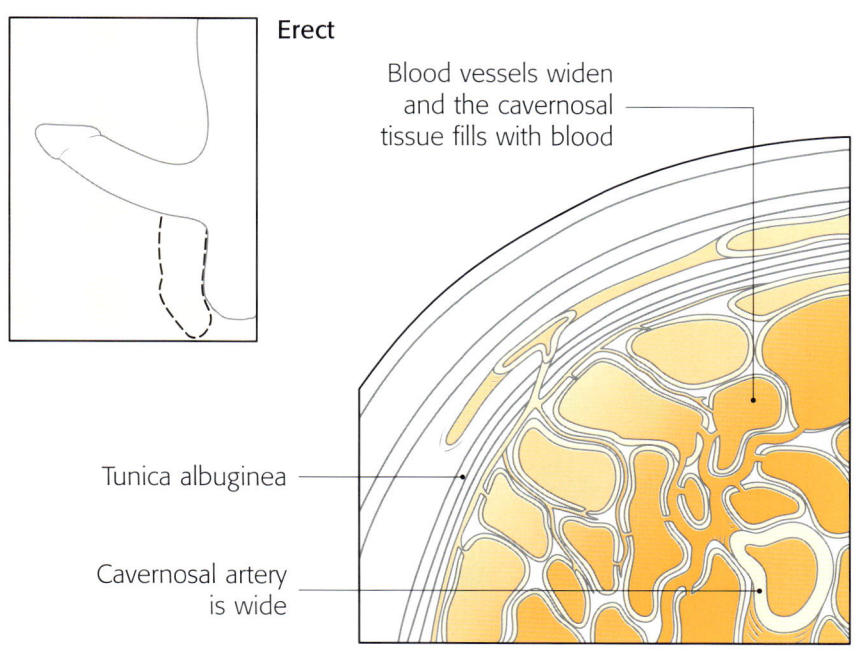

Blood vessels widen and the cavernosal tissue fills with blood

Tunica albuginea

Cavernosal artery is wide

Blood supply and nerve pathways to the penis

- The cavernosal arteries branch from the penile arteries and supply blood to the corpora cavernosa. The cavernosal arteries run down the centre of each corpus cavernosum and divide into twisting (helicine) arteries. These supply blood directly to the erectile tissue.

- The glans at the tip of the penis is supplied with blood from the dorsal artery and the corpus spongiosum.

- Blood is able to flow freely between the different parts of the penis.

- Following an erection, blood drains from the cavernosal spaces of the penis via the emissary veins, which drain into the deep dorsal vein. The penis becomes limp (flaccid) again.

- An erection is the male body's response to sexually stimulating sights, sounds, thoughts and smells. In the central nervous system, the brain sends messages to the spinal cord to produce an erection. The peripheral nervous system is also involved.

- Another part of the nervous system, the sympathetic pathway, is essential for ejaculation and closing the bladder neck during ejaculation. It also controls the penis when it becomes limp.

- Damage to any of these nerve pathways can lead to problems getting and maintaining an erection. Ejaculation can also be affected.

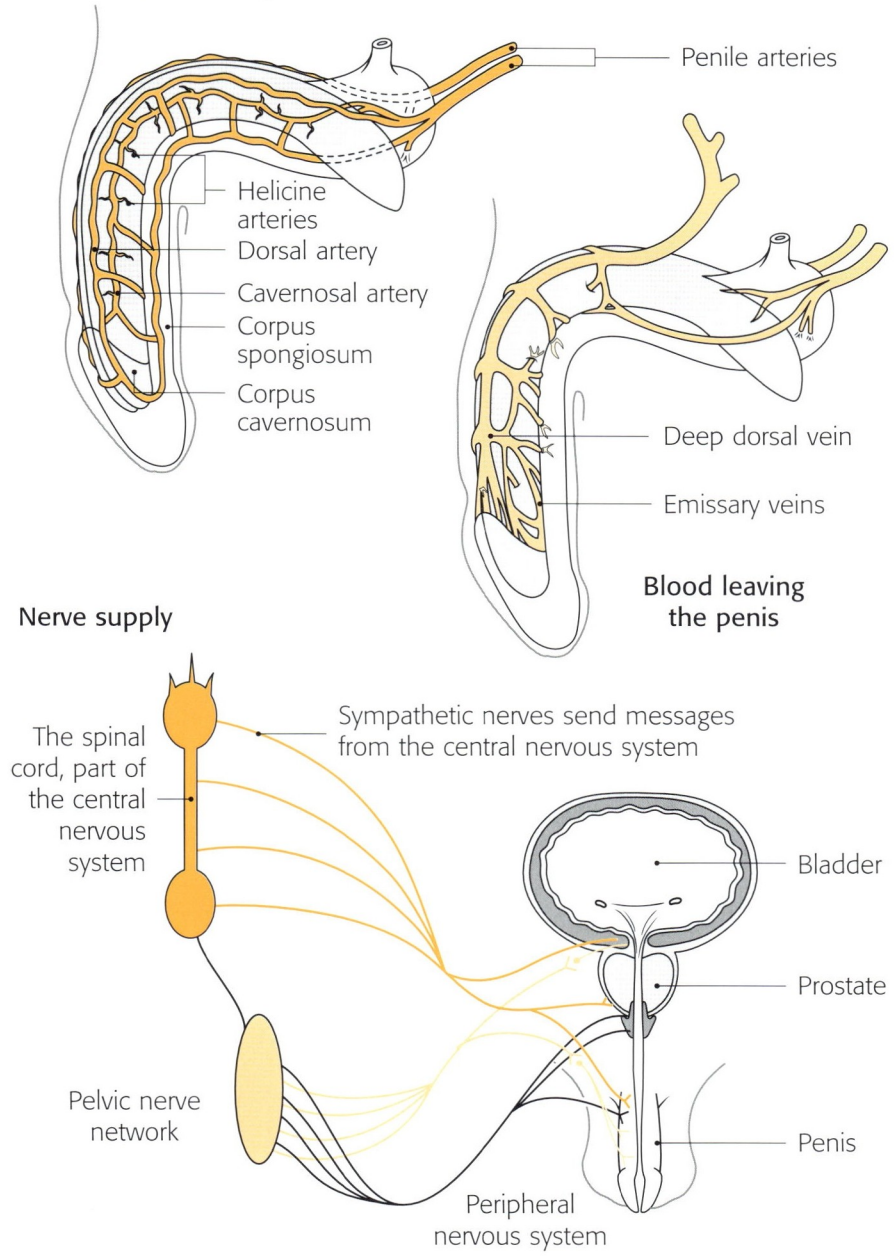

Blood supply to the penis

Penile arteries

Helicine arteries

Dorsal artery

Cavernosal artery

Corpus spongiosum

Corpus cavernosum

Deep dorsal vein

Emissary veins

Blood leaving the penis

Nerve supply

Sympathetic nerves send messages from the central nervous system

The spinal cord, part of the central nervous system

Bladder

Prostate

Pelvic nerve network

Penis

Peripheral nervous system

Biochemical changes during an erection

- For an erection to occur, biochemical changes must take place in a man's body. These changes are the body's response to chemicals released when nerve pathways are stimulated.

- Following sexual stimulation, a chemical messenger called nitric oxide is released from the blood vessels throughout the body, but particularly in the penis.

- Nitric oxide activates other chemical messengers in the smooth muscle of the penis. Some of these chemicals cause the arteries to widen, allowing more blood to enter the penis and an erection to develop.

- An enzyme called phosphodiesterase can stop an erection developing by breaking down one of the chemicals that makes the arteries widen.

- Some treatments for erectile dysfunction (ED) interfere with this biochemical pathway, so sexual stimulation is essential for them to work effectively. Sildenafil (Viagra®), a tablet for the treatment of ED, stops phosphodiesterase working and so keeps a high volume of blood in the penis.

- Erections are a neurovascular event – they are controlled both by the nervous system and blood vessels. This explains why castrated men can still have erections. Male hormones, such as testosterone, do not cause erections. Testosterone is responsible for your sex drive (libido).

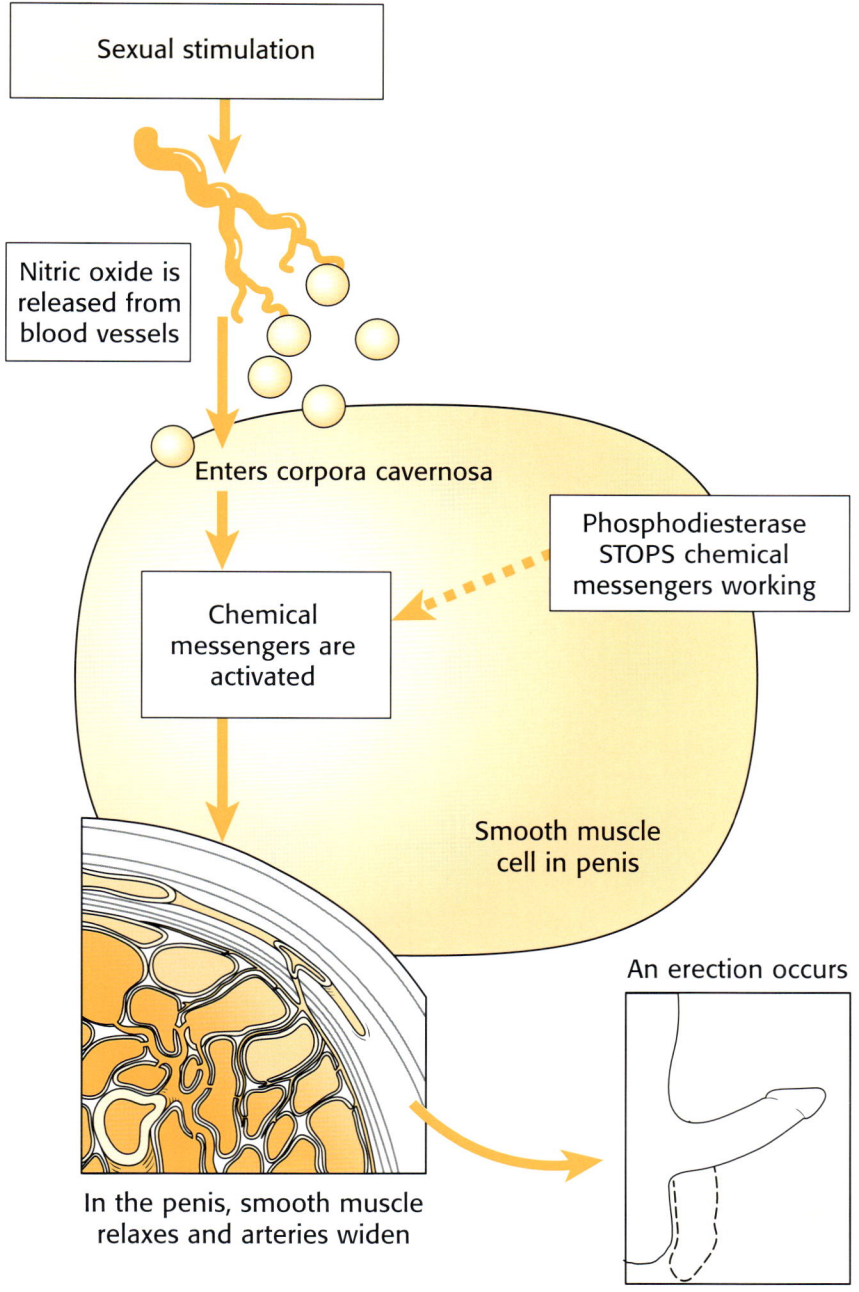

Sexual stimulation

Nitric oxide is released from blood vessels

Enters corpora cavernosa

Phosphodiesterase STOPS chemical messengers working

Chemical messengers are activated

Smooth muscle cell in penis

An erection occurs

In the penis, smooth muscle relaxes and arteries widen

Erectile dysfunction

- Erectile dysfunction (ED) is the consistent inability to get or maintain an erection sufficient to satisfy both you and your sexual partner. Erectile dysfunction is also called impotence.

- At some time, all men experience problems having erections for a variety of reasons, such as stress or excess alcohol intake. This is normal and is not ED.

- You may be able to achieve a short-lived erection that disappears before ejaculation. Because you are unable to maintain your erection, you have ED.

- There is no set length of time that an erection should last. It should simply last long enough to satisfy both you and your partner.

- The Massachusetts Study investigated the link between old age and ED. It showed that, as you get older, you are more likely to have ED. About one-third of men aged 50 years or over have moderate or complete ED. This is probably related to other factors that are more common in men as they get older, such as atherosclerosis (plaques that form in the arteries), rather than being a direct result of ageing.

The Massachusetts data show that as you get older,
you are more likely to have erectile dysfunction

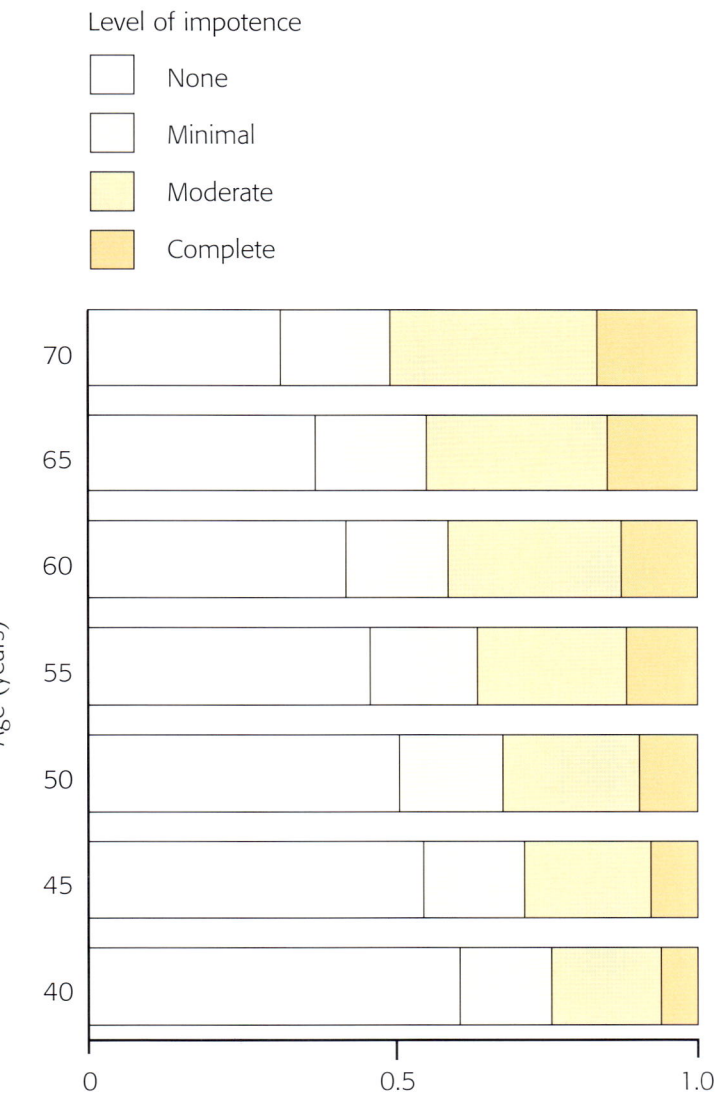

Level of impotence

None

Minimal

Moderate

Complete

Age (years)

Chance of having erectile dysfunction

Medical history

- Your doctor will ask you some questions about your erectile dysfunction (ED). It is important to answer them as fully and honestly as possible if you want to find out the cause of your condition.

- *How long has this been a problem?* Only men who are consistently unable to get and maintain a satisfactory erection need to be assessed and treated. By asking how long you have had the problem, your doctor will know whether or not you have ED.

- *Did the problem begin suddenly or gradually?* If the problem began suddenly and you have not had any pelvic injury or surgery, the cause of your ED is more likely to be psychological than physical.

- *Have you been treated for this problem before?* If previous treatments have been unsuccessful, your doctor will suggest an alternative.

- *Does your partner know that you are coming to speak to me about this problem?* Sexual dysfunction is a problem between a couple, and is neither partner's fault. However, people without a regular sexual partner can still have their ED treated.

- *What do you think has caused this problem?* This will help your doctor to identify specific issues relating to your ED, particularly the psychological aspect.

- *What do you hope to achieve from this consultation?* You may want your doctor to treat your ED. Alternatively, you may not want to discuss treatment options at this stage, but simply want your doctor to make a note of it in your medical records.

- *Do you ejaculate normally?* Tell the doctor whether your ejaculation is normal, premature, delayed or absent.

- *Do you have or have you previously had any diseases?* Some conditions may provide clues to physical problems underlying your ED. For example, tell the doctor if you have diabetes, epilepsy or high blood pressure.

- *Have you had any previous surgery?* Your doctor will be particularly interested in any operations you have had in your pelvic region, such as prostate surgery, or surgery for torsion or undescended testicles.

- *What medications do you or have you previously taken?* Try to remember all the medications that you are currently taking or have taken recently.

- *Do you smoke, drink alcohol or use recreational drugs?* Tell your doctor about your smoking habits, alcohol intake and any recreational drugs you have taken as these can affect sexual function.

Causes of erectile dysfunction

Psychological

- In about 20% of men with erectile dysfunction (ED), the cause is purely psychological. More often, however, ED is due to a combination of psychological and physical factors.

- Psychological factors fall into three categories: predisposing, precipitating and maintaining. Predisposing psychological factors are present before your ED develops, while precipitating factors may bring on your ED initially. Maintaining psychological factors make ED more difficult to overcome in the long term.

- Predisposing factors include an upbringing that associated guilt with sexuality, previous traumatic sexual experiences, disturbed family relationships, and anxiety and stress about work or money.

- Depression, anxiety and loss of a partner may precipitate ED, as can fear of poor sexual performance.

- Once you have ED, this can lead to further anxiety about sexual performance. A lack of communication with or loss of interest in your partner, or a fear of intimacy may also contribute. These are maintaining factors.

Physical

- These may be present from birth (congenital), or related to the nervous system (neurological), hormones (endocrine), blood vessels (vascular) or tissue damage (traumatic).

- Your doctor will ask you some specific questions to find out if other factors, such as ageing, medications or smoking, are responsible for your ED.

- Ageing with atherosclerosis (plaques in the blood vessels that reduce blood flow) is the most common cause of physical ED. Atherosclerosis is associated with smoking.

- Half of all men with diabetes have ED because of damage to their nervous system called autonomic neuropathy, in which the part of the nervous system essential for erections degenerates. Retrograde ejaculation (when semen passes into the bladder) sometimes occurs before ED is apparent.

- Three-quarters of men with chronic renal failure have ED. Many find that their ED improves following a kidney transplant.

Drugs

- In up to a quarter of patients, ED can be a direct result of drugs prescribed to treat other conditions. However, never stop taking medication without first consulting your doctor.

- Medications that cause ED include some antidepressants, drugs to treat high blood pressure, and hormones, such as antiandrogens, oestrogens and LHRH analogues for the treatment of prostate cancer. Other drugs that can cause ED include cimetidine, phenytoin and metoclopramide.

- Alcohol, smoking and recreational drugs, such as marijuana, can cause ED. Any damage can be lasting.

Examination

- If you have erectile dysfunction (ED), your doctor or nurse practitioner will give you a general examination.

- Your penis and testicles will be examined. If your testicles are very small (hypogonadism), they may not be functioning properly.

- If your penis appears to be bent or the opening is on the underside of the penis (hypospadias), this may be related to your condition. However, ED is not related to the length of your penis.

- A swollen scrotum, usually due to an accumulation of watery liquid (a hydrocele) or a large hernia, may envelope your penis, making it difficult to have erections.

- Erections do not depend on male hormones. However, enlarged breasts (gynaecomastia) are evidence of either a chromosome abnormality or a high level of a hormone called prolactin in your blood, which may be related to your ED.

- Your blood pressure will be measured. Your doctor will also check for leg pulses. If these are absent, your blood vessels may have narrowed (atherosclerosis), which can affect your ability to have erections. The central nervous system will also be examined briefly.

- If you are over 50 years of age, you may be given a digital rectal examination as part of routine screening to check your prostate gland.

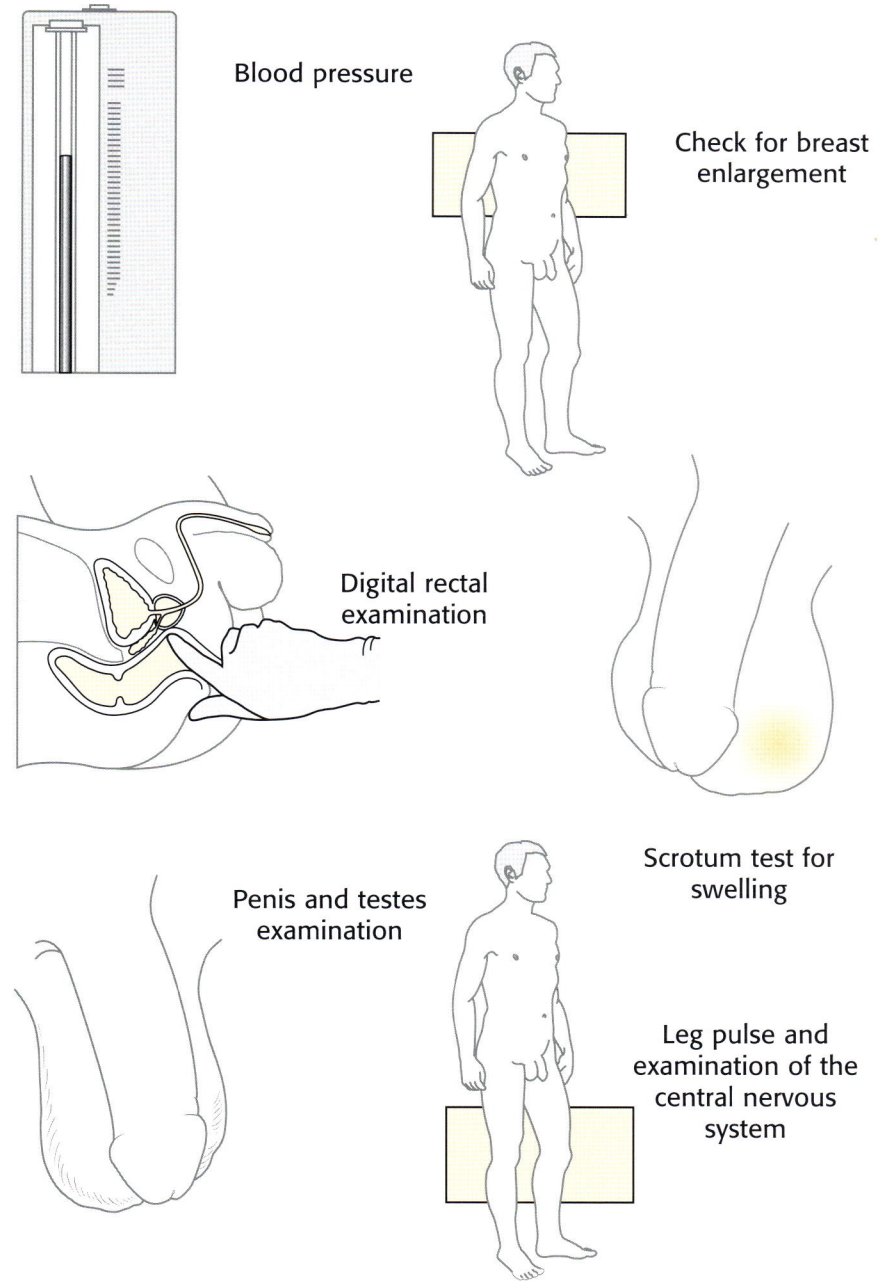

Blood pressure

Check for breast enlargement

Digital rectal examination

Scrotum test for swelling

Penis and testes examination

Leg pulse and examination of the central nervous system

© Health Press Limited

Investigations

- As part of your general examination, your urine will be tested for glucose. If the level is high, you may have diabetes, which may be the cause of your erectile dysfunction (ED). A blood test will confirm the diagnosis.

- Hormone levels in your blood may also be tested. Although erections do not depend on hormones, low testosterone can reduce your sex drive. Your doctor can prescribe treatment to increase your testosterone. If your testosterone is low, a full hormone screen will be performed to look for any other abnormalities.

- To check the blood supply to your penis, your doctor will inject a vasoactive drug (alprostadil) directly into the penis to widen the arteries and increase the blood flow. The needle is small and the injection is not painful, though it may be a little uncomfortable. If a satisfactory erection develops, the blood supply to your penis is sufficient and not the reason for your ED.

- If you do not have an erection following the injection, the blood supply to your penis is inadequate. Further tests will help your doctor determine the best treatment for you.

- Injections directly into the penis can also show deformities, such as Peyronie's disease (fibrous plaques that make the penis bend) and curvature. Photographs and measurements of your erect penis may be taken as a record of your condition. Your penis can then be compared before and after treatment.

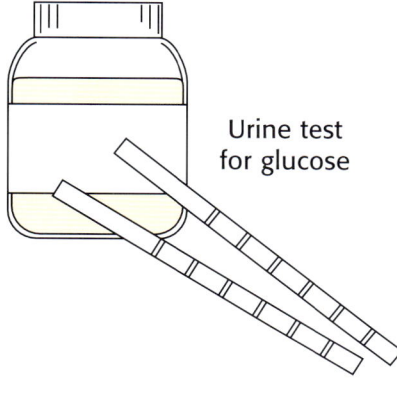

Urine test for glucose

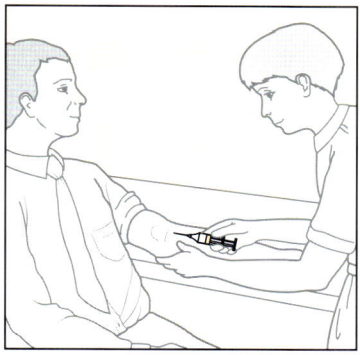

Blood test

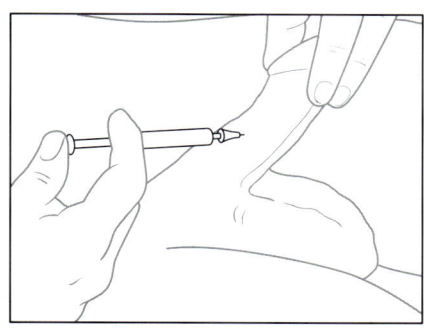

Injecting a vasoactive drug directly into the penis will check the blood flow and show deformities

Photographs and measurements provide a record of your condition

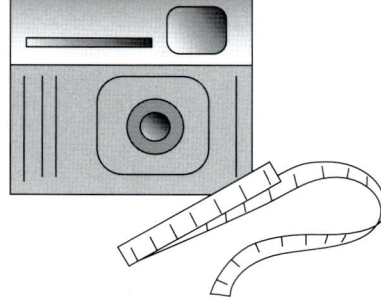

Night-time erections (nocturnal penile tumescences)

- While sleeping, men normally have three or four erections a night, each lasting for up to 20 minutes. These occur during periods of rapid eye movement sleep and are called nocturnal penile tumescences (NPTs).

- If your erectile dysfunction (ED) is caused by psychological factors, you are still likely to have NPTs. However, if your ED is due to physical factors, you will not. Testing whether or not you have NPTs will help identify the cause of your ED.

- A simple but effective test is the stamp test. Before going to bed, place a strip of stamps around the penis. If a good erection occurs during the night, the perforations will snap.

- The RigiScan® is a more sophisticated device that allows continuous night-time monitoring. It is very easy to use. Two rings are placed around the penis, one at the base and the other around the shaft. The rings measure changes in the girth of the penis every 30 seconds and changes in firmness or rigidity every 3 minutes. A rigidity of more than 75% means that your erections are satisfactory.

- For the tests to work properly, you must sleep normally. It is therefore best to do the tests at home on 1 or 2 nights.

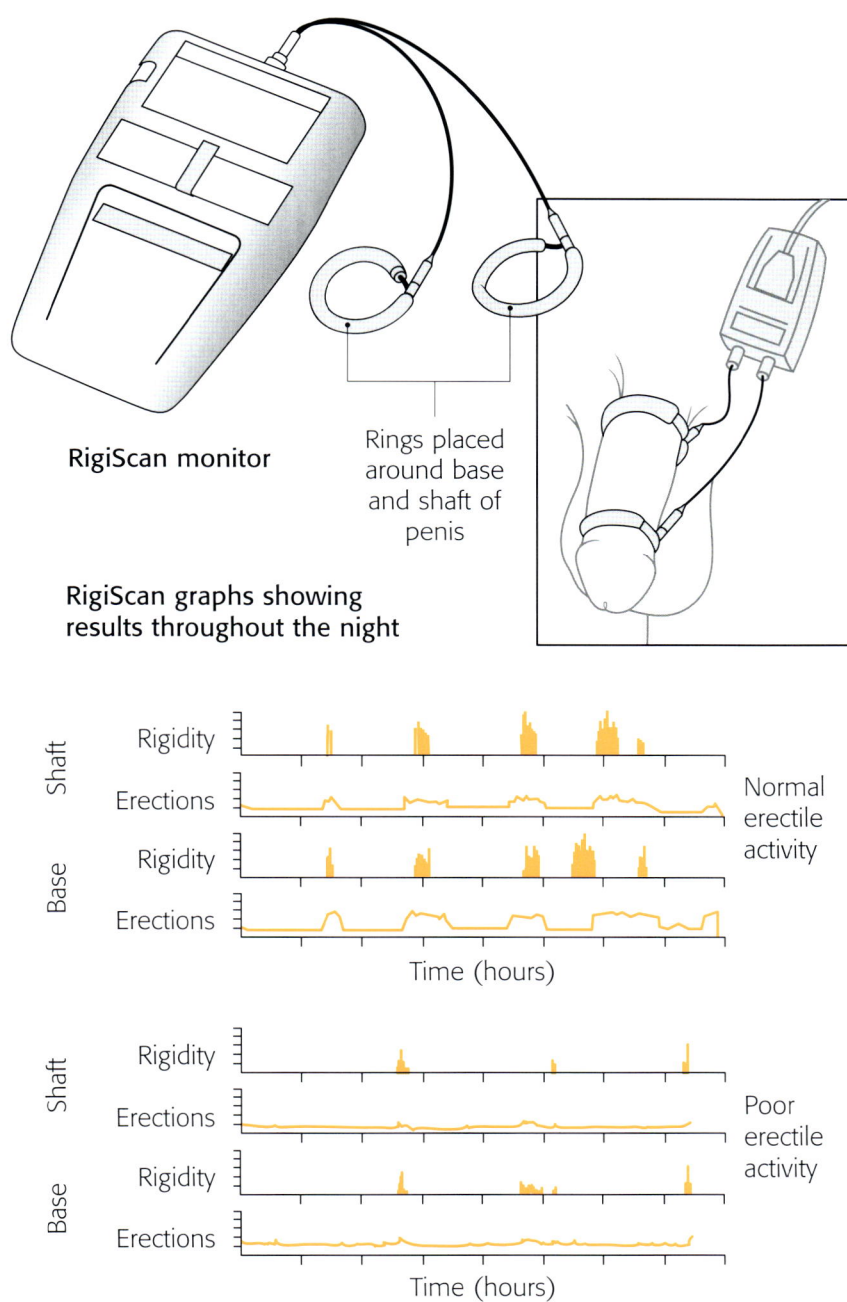

RigiScan monitor

Rings placed around base and shaft of penis

RigiScan graphs showing results throughout the night

Shaft — Rigidity / Erections

Base — Rigidity / Erections

Time (hours)

Normal erectile activity

Shaft — Rigidity / Erections

Base — Rigidity / Erections

Time (hours)

Poor erectile activity

Colour Doppler ultrasonography

- If you do not have a satisfactory erection following an intrapenile injection with a vasoactive drug (alprostadil), a special type of scan (colour Doppler ultrasonography) can show if the blood flow to the penis is too low. In colour Doppler ultrasonography, changes in ultrasound frequencies provide information about the blood flow.

- This technique is particularly useful if your pelvic area has been injured. It will show if the blood supply to your penis has been damaged. If it has, it may be possible to correct this by reconstructive surgery.

- Colour Doppler ultrasonography is not painful. Alprostadil is injected directly into the penis with a small needle to produce an erection. A gel is applied to the penis and an ultrasound probe is used to glide across its surface. The blood vessels are scanned from the base to the tip for up to 30 minutes after the injection.

- A graph on the computer screen will indicate whether or not the blood flow to your penis is adequate.

- Colour Doppler ultrasonography may show that blood is leaking from the veins in the penis, preventing it from staying rigid. Further investigations are necessary to confirm this.

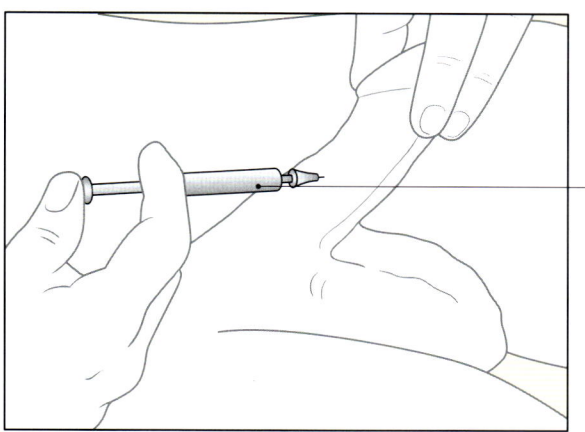

Colour Doppler ultrasonography

Vasoactive injection to increase the blood flow and produce an erection

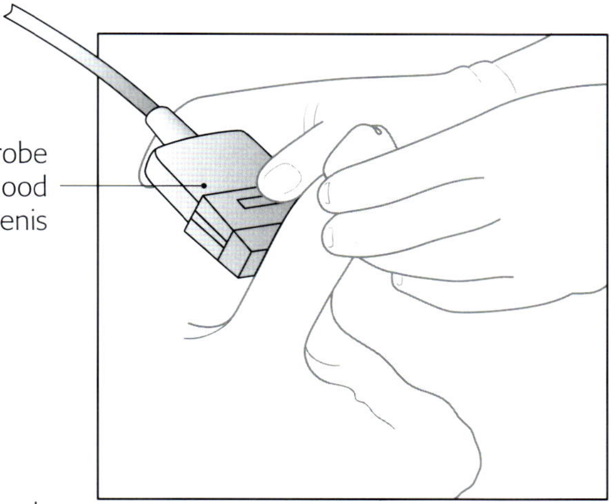

Ultrasound probe scans the blood vessels of the penis

A colour Doppler graph showing normal peak blood flow during an erection

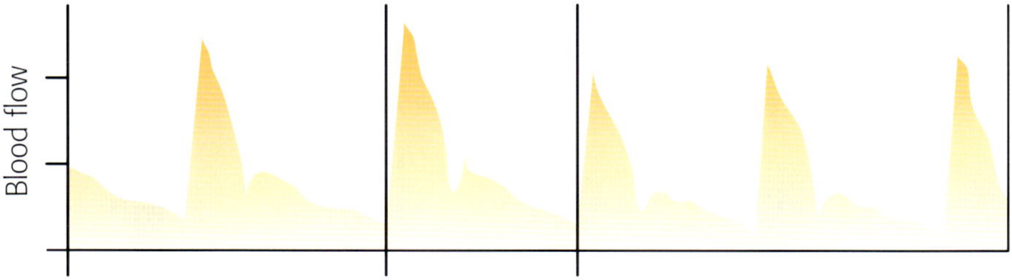

Blood flow

Cavernosometry and cavernosography

- Young men who can have but not maintain erections may have venous leakage. This reduces pressure in the penis and stops it from staying rigid. Venous leakage can be confirmed using a special type of scan (colour Doppler ultrasonography) followed by cavernosography.

- Cavernosometry is an important investigation in erectile dysfunction, and is used to measure the blood flow rate necessary to produce and maintain an erection.

- While you are lying down, two very small needles (butterfly needles) are inserted into the penis. This may be uncomfortable, but is not painful. A drug is given through one of the needles to widen the blood vessels and cause an erection, followed by a saline infusion, which allows the pressure to be measured through the second needle.

- A machine measures the flow rates needed to achieve and maintain an erection. The pressure is shown as a graph, and indicates whether or not the erectile mechanism is working.

- In cavernosography, an X-ray contrast substance is injected into the penis. X-rays are then taken to show any venous leakage. The injection may be a little uncomfortable. If the penis is not fully rigid, venous leakage will occur regardless.

- Cavernosography alone can be used to show space in the corpora following fibrosis after a prolonged erection (priapism) or removal of a penile prosthesis, and also to view plaques in Peyronie's disease.

Cavernosometry

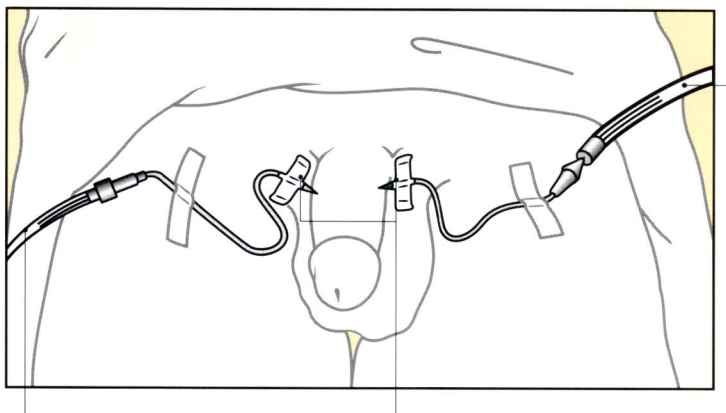

Pressure is measured through the second needle

Vasoactive drug increases blood flow and produces an erection

Butterfly needles in erectile tissue

Cavernosography

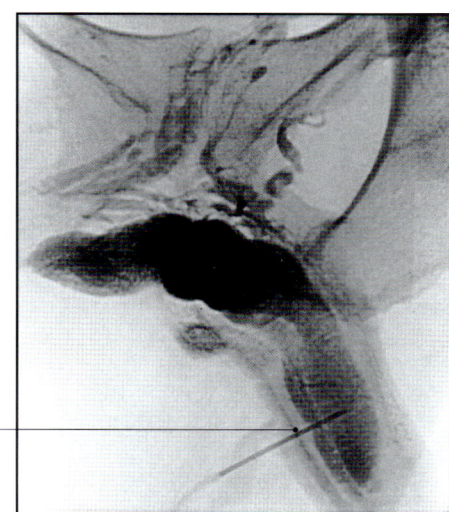

X-ray shows fibrosis (thickened and scarred tissue) in the penis

Psychosexual therapy

- Your doctor may recommend a visit to a psychosexual counsellor to help treat your erectile dysfunction (ED).

- Your counsellor will help you to understand the factors involved in your ED, giving you and your partner the opportunity to discuss and deal with the issues openly.

- Some counsellors recommend sensate focus therapy. At first, no intercourse is allowed. You and your partner are encouraged to undress and touch each other, but not genitally, two or three times a week. Because no intercourse occurs, the fear of failure is removed. When you are both fully relaxed, which may take several weeks, you should stimulate each other genitally and become more comfortable with each other's body. At this stage, you should not proceed to intercourse or orgasm.

- Many men lose their erection at penetration. In the final stage of sensate focus, penetration takes place, but neither partner moves further (vaginal containment). When you can do this without losing your erection, you should proceed to movement, orgasm and ejaculation.

- Other counsellors will suggest a cognitive approach, in which you will be encouraged to deal with the negative thoughts, such as anxiety and fear, that affect your normal sexual function. By confronting these thoughts, you may learn to overcome them.

- During psychosexual therapy, you must be prepared for your counsellor to identify underlying causes that you may be unwilling to confront.

Psychosexual therapy

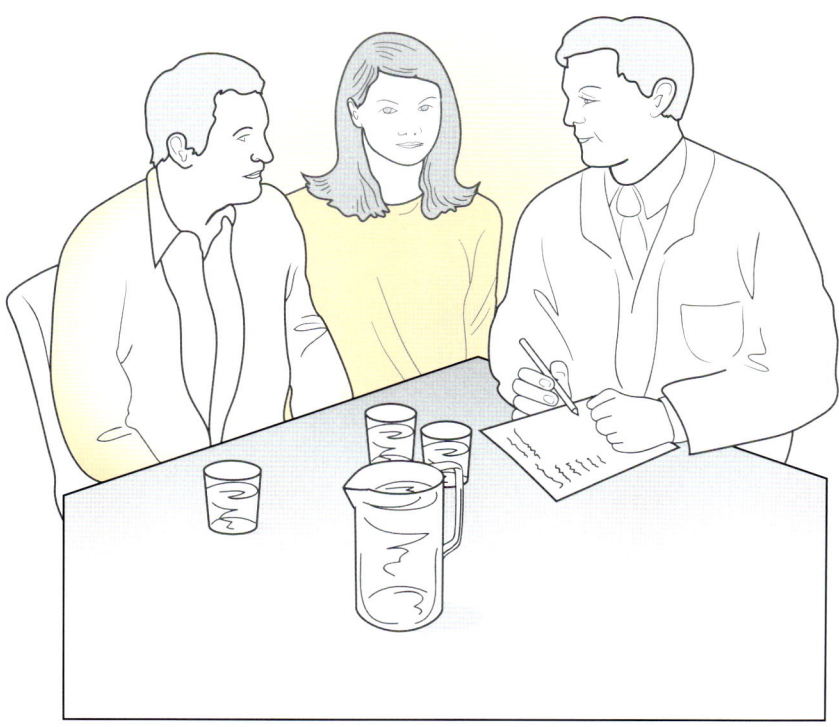

Androgen-replacement therapy

- The testicles secrete testosterone, which controls sex drive (libido). If your testicles are small (hypogonadism), they may not function properly. A blood test will show if your testosterone is low.

- If you have high levels of a hormone called prolactin in your blood, your pituitary gland may not be functioning properly. This is rare, and you will need to be referred to an endocrinologist for treatment.

- Androgens stimulate the development of male sex organs. If your testosterone levels are low, you may be given androgen-replacement therapy as tablets, intramuscular injections every 3–4 weeks, pellets inserted under the skin or skin patches.

- Androgen-replacement therapy side-effects are quite rare, but include general water retention, thickened blood, breast formation, headache, anxiety, acne, excess hair, jaundice, hepatitis and liver cancer.

- There is some evidence that androgen-replacement therapy causes prostate enlargement. Because of this, a digital rectal examination and/or a blood test (prostate-specific antigen level) will be performed every 6 months to check your prostate gland for changes.

- You cannot have androgen-replacement therapy if you already have prostate cancer because androgen makes cancer cells grow.

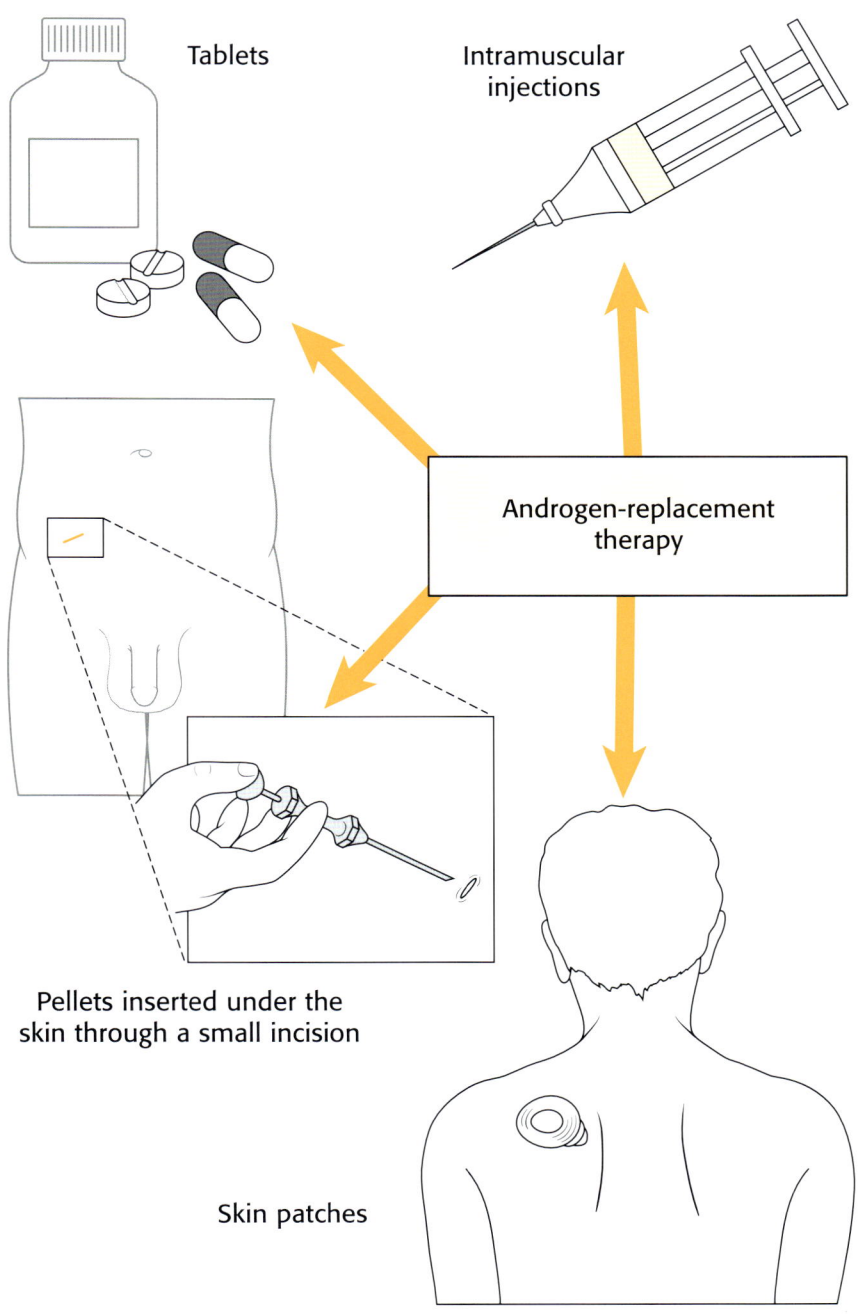

Tablets

Intramuscular injections

Androgen-replacement therapy

Pellets inserted under the skin through a small incision

Skin patches

Oral treatment

- There are a number of different tablets that can be taken to treat erectile dysfunction (ED). Each works in a different way.

- If your ED does not have a physical cause, yohimbine, a plant extract, may improve your sex drive (libido). Side-effects include palpitations, a frequent need to pass urine, nausea, indigestion and headaches, but these will pass.

- Trazodone, an antidepressant, is an effective treatment for ED in some men. It may cause a number of side-effects, such as a dry mouth, an inability to pass urine, constipation and blurred vision. These side-effects will disappear when you stop taking trazodone.

- Sildenafil (Viagra®) is an effective oral treatment for ED. It must be taken approximately 1 hour before sexual intercourse is expected to take place and will produce an erection only if you are stimulated sexually. You must not take sildenafil if you are taking nitrates for angina.

- Other new oral treatments are likely to be available soon – your doctor can tell you about these.

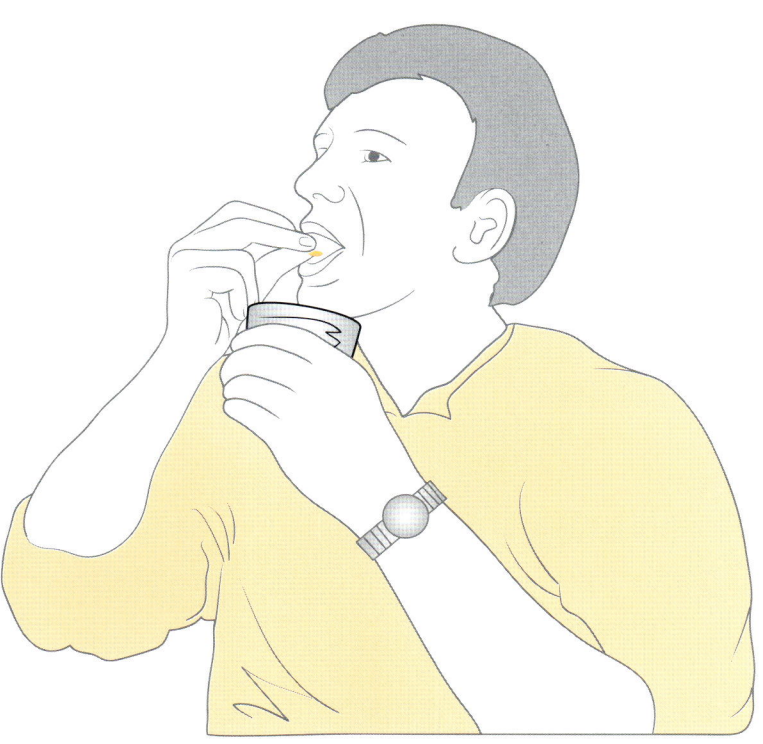

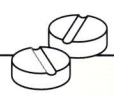

Oral treatments for erectile dysfunction

- Yohimbine – a plant extract

- Trazodone – an antidepressant

- Sildenafil – works only if you are sexually stimulated

Sildenafil: how it works

- Following sexual stimulation, blood vessels release nitric oxide. This activates chemical messengers, including cGMP, that increase the blood flow to the penis.

- An enzyme, phosphodiesterase, breaks down cGMP. Sildenafil (Viagra®), a tablet for erectile dysfunction, stops phosphodiesterase working, keeping a high blood flow to the penis.

- Sildenafil must never be taken if you are also taking nitrates, which are often prescribed for angina, because this can lead to a life-threatening drop in blood pressure. Also, you must never use the recreational drug amyl nitrate (poppers) with sildenafil.

- Common side-effects of sildenafil are headaches, facial flushing, heartburn and a blocked nose. These occur in 3–10% of patients. Rarely, patients complain of changes in their colour perception, but this soon passes.

- Sildenafil is removed mainly from the body by a liver enzyme. Some drugs – such as cimetidine, ketoconazole, erythromycin and the protease inhibitors used to treat HIV – stop this enzyme working and may prevent sildenafil being removed from your body quickly. If you are taking medication that stops this enzyme working, you will need to take a lower dose of sildenafil so that levels do not build up in your body.

- You will usually be given a 50 mg dose of sildenafil to start with. If this does not work, the dose can be increased to 100 mg. In young patients, 25 mg is probably sufficient to give a satisfactory erection.

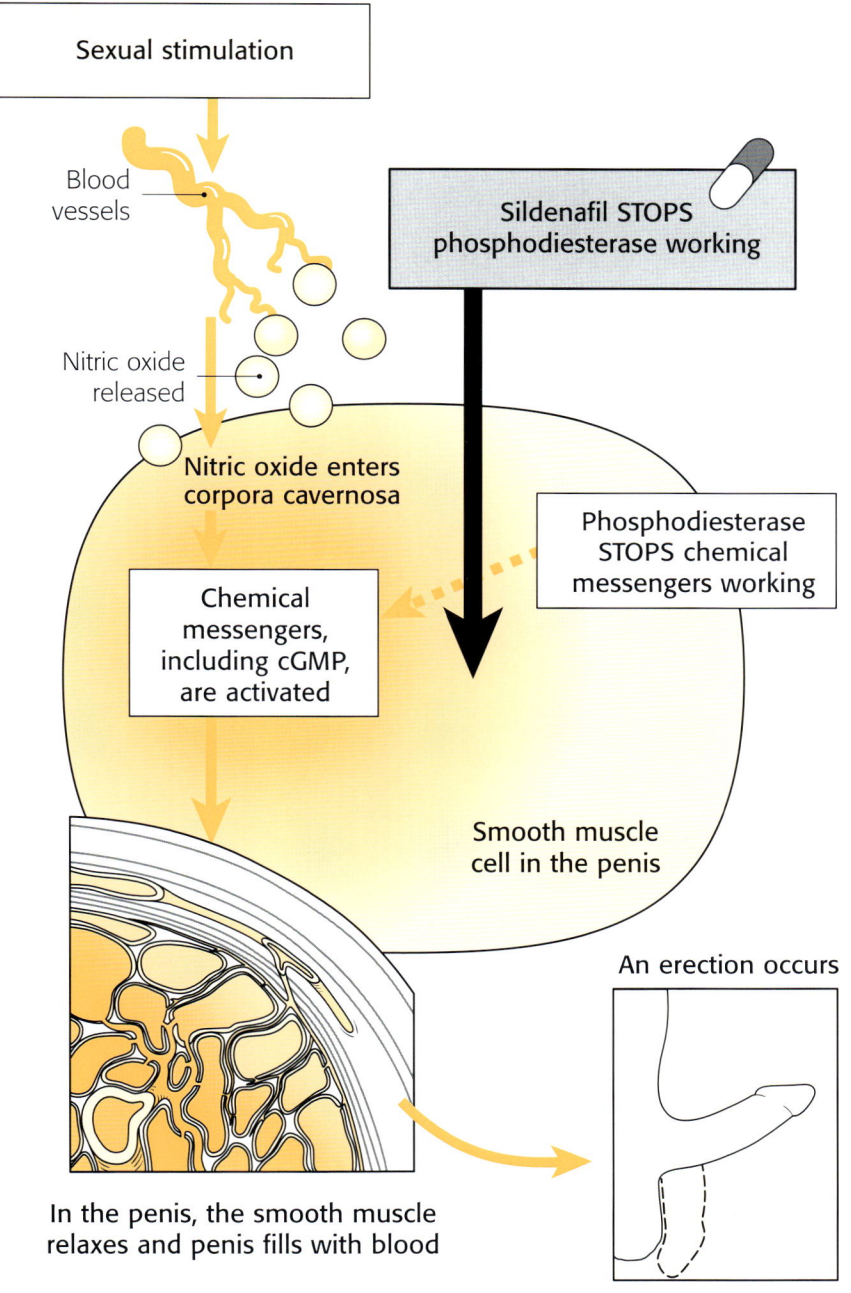

Sexual stimulation

Blood vessels

Sildenafil STOPS phosphodiesterase working

Nitric oxide released

Nitric oxide enters corpora cavernosa

Phosphodiesterase STOPS chemical messengers working

Chemical messengers, including cGMP, are activated

Smooth muscle cell in the penis

An erection occurs

In the penis, the smooth muscle relaxes and penis fills with blood

Sildenafil: who can take it

- Sildenafil (Viagra®) is an effective oral treatment for erectile dysfunction (ED). It can also improve your orgasm and sexual satisfaction. Often, your sexual partner will also notice an improvement in your erection.

- If your ED is due to psychological or nerve-related problems, high blood pressure or depression, sildenafil is particularly effective. About half the patients who have had surgery for prostate enlargement, such as radical prostatectomy or pelvic surgery, find that sildenafil treats their ED successfully.

- It is important to remember sildenafil is not an aphrodisiac and does not increase sexual desire.

- Sildenafil should be taken approximately 1 hour before you expect sexual intercourse to take place. Because of the way in which sildenafil works, you will only have an erection if you are stimulated sexually.

- If you have coronary artery disease, you must be able to walk a mile in 20 minutes and then climb two flights of stairs to be fit enough to have sexual intercourse. If you cannot do this, you will need to discuss your situation with your doctor in more detail.

- Sildenafil must never be taken if you are also taking nitrates, which are often prescribed for angina, as this can lead to a life-threatening drop in blood pressure.

Sildenafil is not suitable for all types of erectile dysfunction

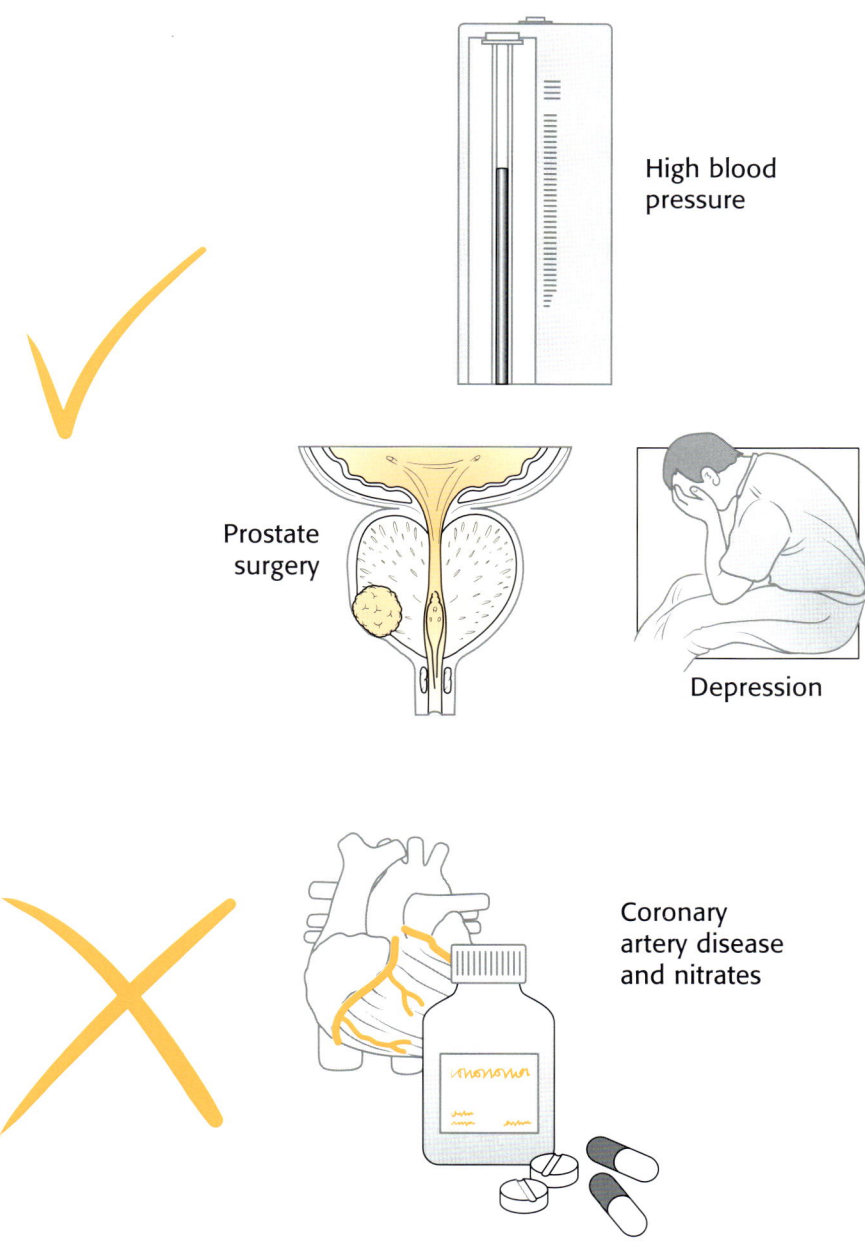

High blood pressure

Prostate surgery

Depression

Coronary artery disease and nitrates

Intracavernosal therapy

- Injecting a vasoactive drug, which relaxes blood vessels and increases blood flow, directly into the erectile tissue of the penis (intracavernosal injection) produces an erection. This is a very effective treatment for erectile dysfunction (ED).

- Intracavernosal therapy (Caverject®, Caverject® Dual Chamber, Viridal® Duo) is particularly useful for ED due to damage to the nervous system. It can also be of benefit if oral treatment is unsuccessful, or if you want to know if your ED is caused by a reduced blood flow.

- Intracavernosal therapy is easy to use. However, the need for an injection means there is a lack of spontaneity in sexual relations, so it is not ideal for everyone.

- Intracavernosal therapy produces stronger and more predictable erections than other treatments for ED.

- Alprostadil is the most frequently prescribed vasoactive drug. Following the first injection, about one-third of patients experience a spontaneous improvement in their erections as if their erectile mechanism has 'woken up'.

- Your nurse or doctor will administer your first injection. While lying down, you will be given an injection, which is not painful, into the side of the penis near the base, away from the midline. It will take about 5 minutes for an erection to develop fully. The firmness of the erection can be compared with previous ones, and the dose adjusted appropriately.

Intracavernosal therapy

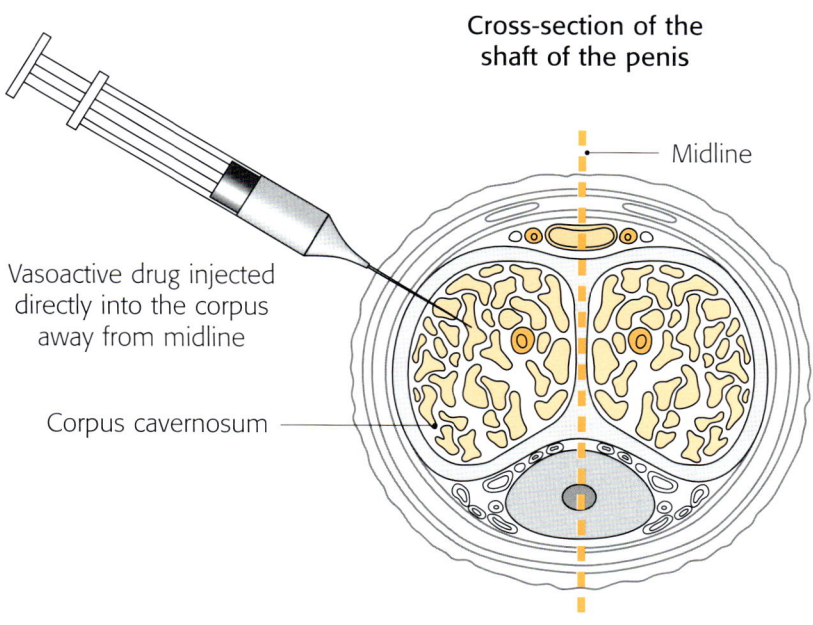

Midline

Injection sites for intracavernosal therapy

Deep dorsal vein

Cross-section of the shaft of the penis

Midline

Vasoactive drug injected directly into the corpus away from midline

Corpus cavernosum

Self-administering intracavernosal therapy

- Your doctor or nurse will show you how to prepare the alprostadil injection. While sitting down, hold the tip (glans) of your penis between your thumb and index finger, and position it towards your thigh. Hold the needle and syringe at a right angle to the penis. Inject near the base of the penis, away from the midline and avoiding any visible veins. Compress the injection site for 1 minute.

- The needle is small, so the injection is not usually painful. A burning pain from the drug itself can occur in a small percentage of patients, and may last for 1–2 hours; this improves with repeated use. If any bruising or bleeding occurs, check with your doctor that you are injecting correctly.

- If you have an unsteady hand because of multiple sclerosis, Parkinson's disease or a stroke, a willing partner can be taught to inject.

- If you have a good erection following your first intra-cavernosal injection, there is a small risk of prolonged erection (priapism). If your erection remains after 3 hours, you will need to take a terbutaline tablet, which is distributed in some clinics. If the erection lasts more than 4 hours, go to the local clinic or casualty <u>immediately</u>, indicating the treatment you have used and when.

- Thickening (fibrosis) of the erectile tissue may occur even after using intracavernosal therapy successfully for some time. If this happens, stop injecting immediately and consult your doctor. As you get older, you may find that the effect of intracavernosal therapy is gradually lost.

Self-administering intracavernosal therapy

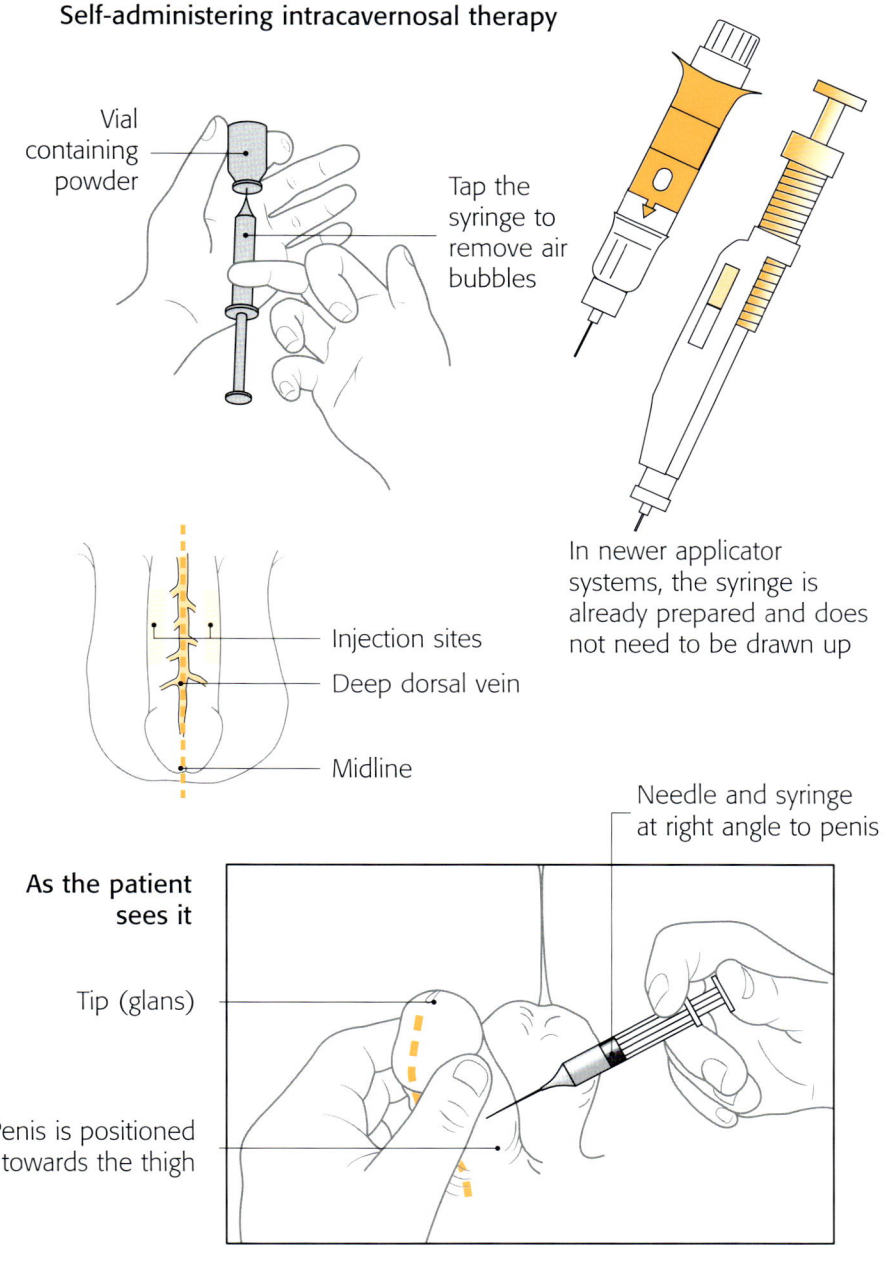

Vial containing powder

Tap the syringe to remove air bubbles

In newer applicator systems, the syringe is already prepared and does not need to be drawn up

Injection sites

Deep dorsal vein

Midline

Needle and syringe at right angle to penis

As the patient sees it

Tip (glans)

Penis is positioned towards the thigh

Intraurethral drug delivery

- If the blood flow to your penis is inadequate, a vasoactive drug can increase the blood flow and produce an erection. The drug can be inserted directly into the urethra through the opening at the end of the penis and then absorbed into the rest of the penis (MUSE®, Medicated Urethral System for Erection).

- A specially designed plastic applicator is used to insert a pellet of alprostadil, a vasoactive drug, into the urethra.

- One- to two-thirds of men achieve an erection adequate for sex with intraurethral therapy. It is ideal if you dislike injections, have an unsteady hand or are overweight.

- Before inserting the applicator, you need to urinate to lubricate the urethra and to make it easier for the drug to dissolve. The applicator is placed in the urethra and the button depressed to release the pellet. The device is removed, and the penis massaged gently. After 10 minutes, you should develop an erection that will last about 30 minutes. The dose can be adjusted depending on the firmness of your erection.

- About one-third of men experience mild burning following intraurethral administration. Occasionally, female partners will have vaginal discomfort.

- A constriction ring can improve erections with intraurethral therapy. It is an adjustable lasso-shaped piece of latex that is placed around the base of the penis to prevent blood leaving. The ring should not remain in place for more than 30 minutes as this can damage the tissues in the penis.

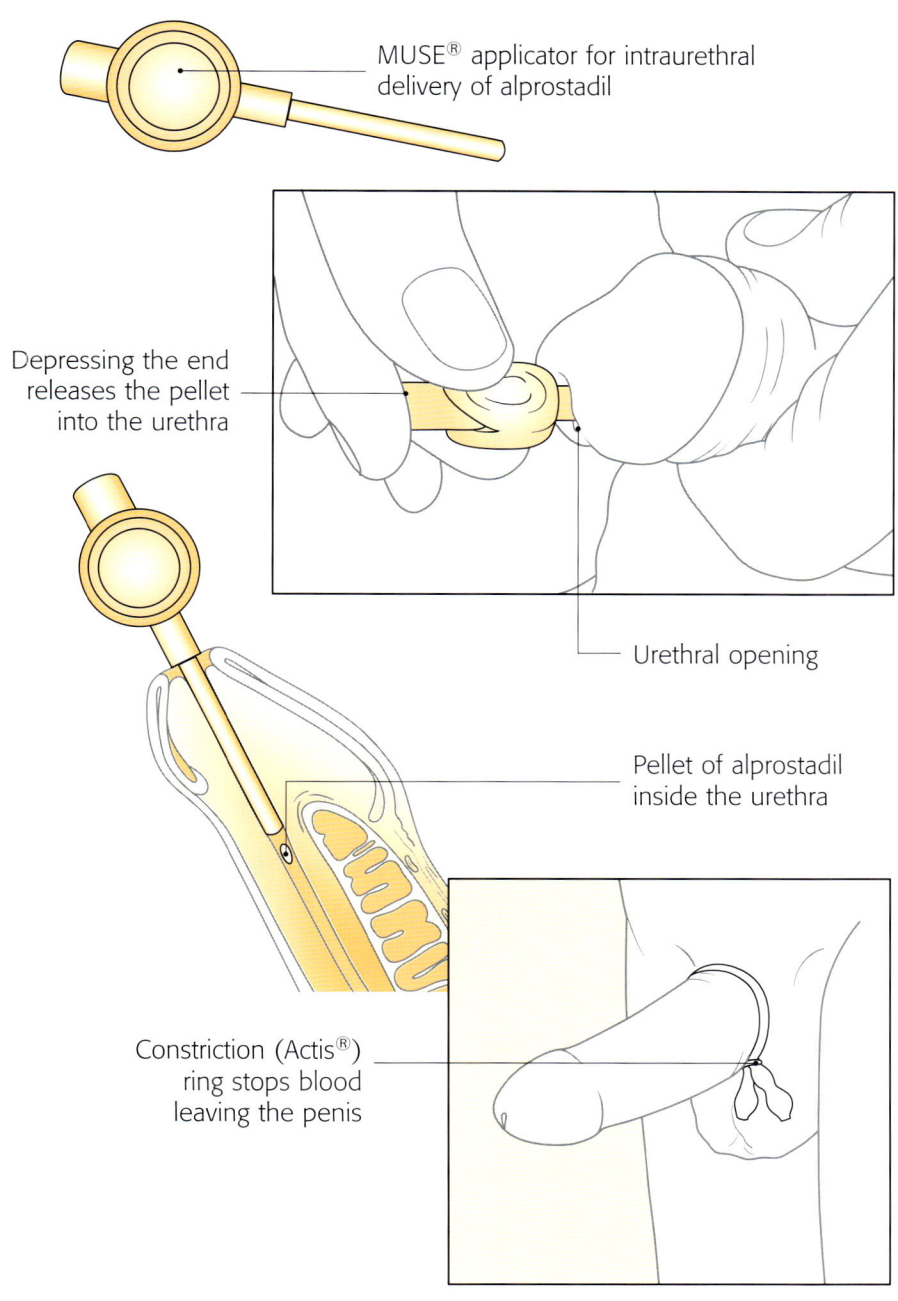

MUSE® applicator for intraurethral delivery of alprostadil

Depressing the end releases the pellet into the urethra

Urethral opening

Pellet of alprostadil inside the urethra

Constriction (Actis®) ring stops blood leaving the penis

Monitoring your treatment

- To assess how effective your treatment for erectile dysfunction (ED) has been, your doctor might ask you to keep a record of your erections.

- In your diary, you should keep a note each time you use your treatment to get an erection. Make a record of the date and the treatment you used. You will need to answer some questions about your erection – how strong or firm it was, how long it lasted and how pleased you were with it. You will also need to list any side-effects you experienced.

- You can describe the strength of your erection using a scale of 1 to 4. If your penis is only slightly swollen, you will record the strength of erection as grade 1. Grade 2 describes swelling of the penis insufficient for penetrative sex, while Grade 3 is firm enough for penetration but not a full erection. If you have a full, stiff erection that is sufficient for penetrative sex, this should be recorded as grade 4.

- Using a similar scale, you should rate how pleased you and your partner were with the result. If you were not happy with the result, you will write down 1. If you were delighted with the result, you should write 4.

- Take your diary with you when you visit your doctor. You can discuss how successful you feel your treatment has been. If you are not happy with the results, your doctor can recommend an alternative therapy. You may need to try more than one type of treatment before you find the one that is best for you.

A treatment diary

Date	Treatment	Strength of erection	Side-effects	How long?	Were you pleased?	Satis-faction
7/2/00	name of treatment	4	none	30 min	3	4

Topical treatment

- Topical vasoactive drugs can be applied directly onto the penis to increase blood flow and improve erections. Topical preparations are available as gels, ointments, solutions and patches, and can be applied when needed.

- Although topical drugs are not used widely for erectile dysfunction, they are moderately successful at producing erections. They are particularly good if you have a spinal injury because the blood supply to your penis will be unaffected and application is easy.

- Most topical preparations need to be applied approximately 1 hour before sexual intercourse. If a patch is used, it should be removed after an hour.

- The most effective topical drug is minoxidil. Other available treatments include nitroglycerin patches and ointment, vasoactive intestinal polypeptide ointment, alprostadil gel and papaverine gel.

- The only side-effect associated with topical preparations is headache. If your treatment gives you a headache, you should stop using it and return to your doctor.

22

Topical treatment

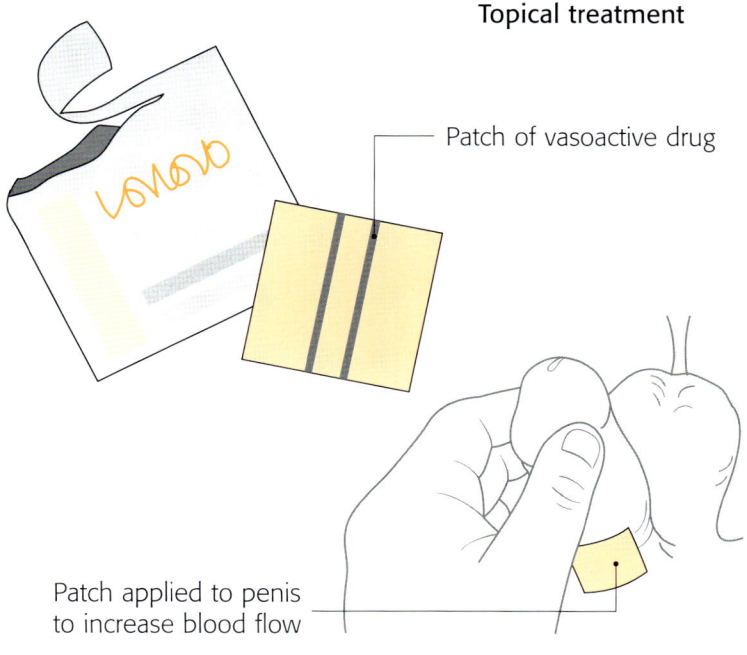

Patch of vasoactive drug

Patch applied to penis
to increase blood flow

Ointments and gels
should be applied to
the whole penis

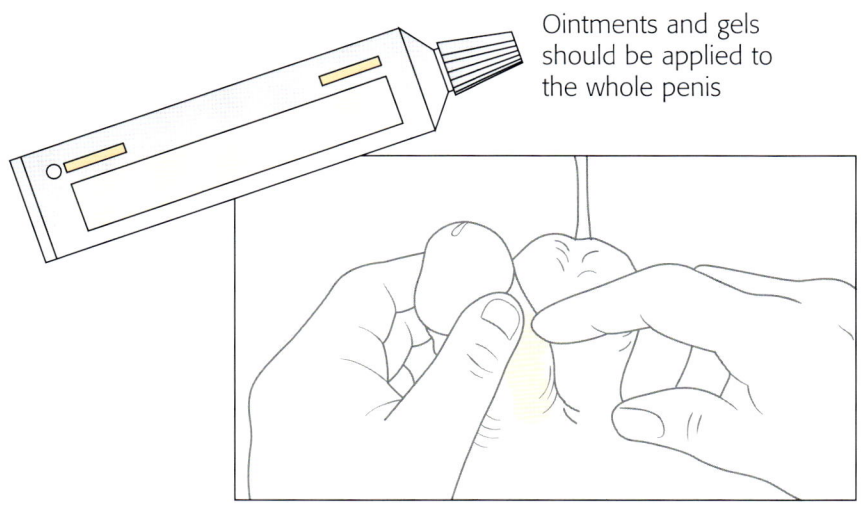

Vacuum devices

- Vacuum devices are an effective, non-invasive treatment for erectile dysfunction (ED) and are suitable for most men. Creating a negative pressure around the penis increases the blood flow to the penis. A constriction ring applied to the base of the penis maintains the erection.

- A vacuum device consists of a vacuum chamber, with a constriction ring applied, and a hand- or battery-operated pump. It produces a satisfactory erection within a few minutes.

- Vacuum devices have very few side-effects other than bruising, and are therefore a safe treatment option. The constriction ring must be removed after 30 minutes to prevent damage to the tissues in the penis.

- Your orgasm will be normal, but your ejaculate (sperm and semen) may be trapped behind the constriction ring. A vacuum device is therefore not suitable if you are trying to get your partner pregnant.

- As vacuum devices are not available on the NHS, you will need to buy one. They are supplied with instructions and a video. Before deciding the device is of no use, try it for at least a month. Many clinics will be able to lend you the equipment to try first.

- Vacuum devices can remove the spontaneity from sexual relations. They can also be fiddly and a bit unsightly, but with continued use, they become easier. Patients in long-term relationships with understanding partners will benefit most from vacuum devices.

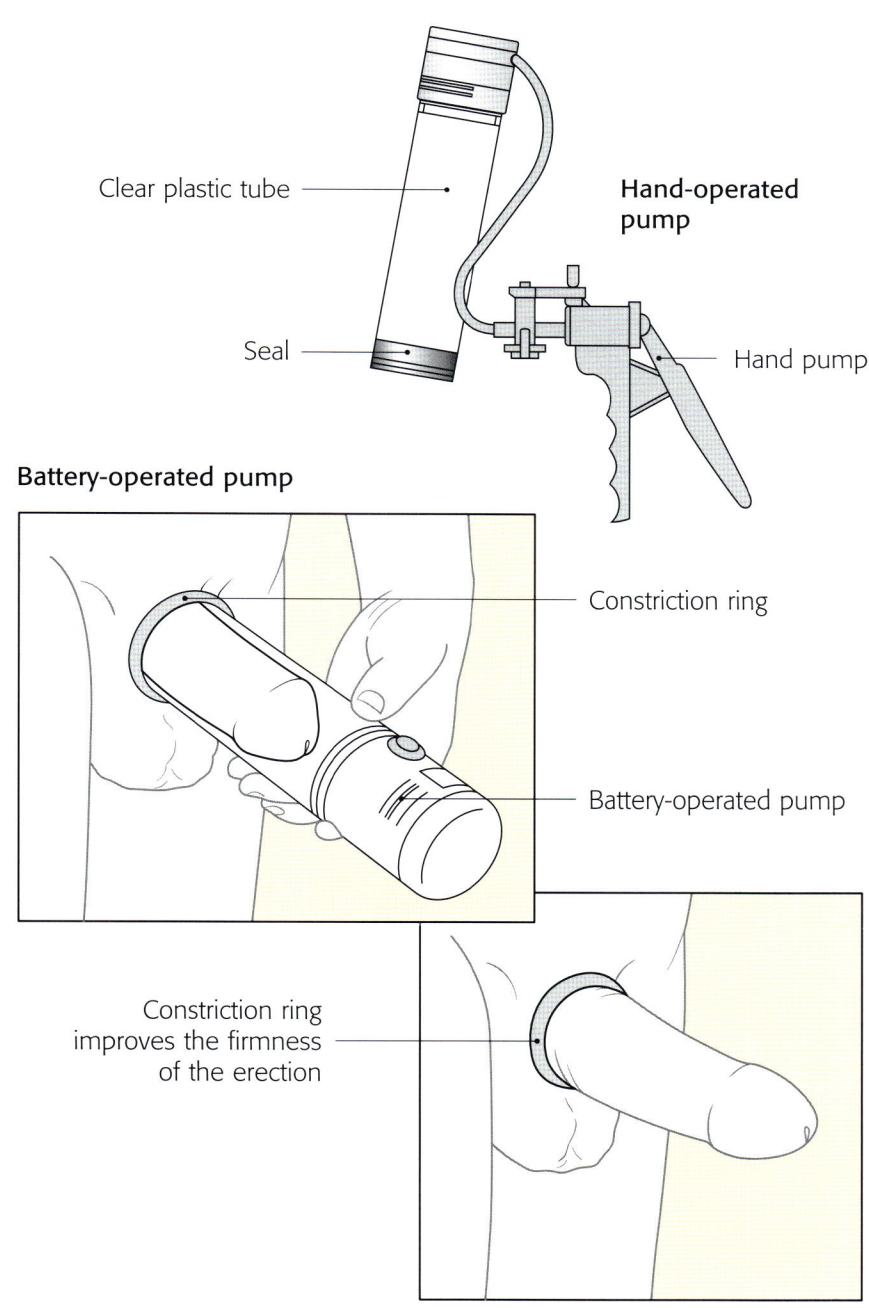

23

Clear plastic tube

Hand-operated pump

Seal

Hand pump

Battery-operated pump

Constriction ring

Battery-operated pump

Constriction ring improves the firmness of the erection

Penile prostheses

- A penile prosthesis is an artificial rod inserted surgically into the penis. It is the final option when all other erectile dysfunction treatments have failed.

- A prosthesis may benefit patients with fibrosis (thickening) following intracavernosal therapy, Peyronie's disease (a fibrous plaque that causes the penis to bend) or an untreated prolonged erection (priapism).

- Three types are available; semi-rigid malleable rods, inflatable cylinders and multi-part inflatable prostheses. Your doctor will discuss the surgical options with you. The semi-rigid rod protrudes and may be embarrassing, while an inflatable three-piece is expensive, but can be pumped up and down. It is important to understand that a prosthesis can never fully replace the erection you had when you were younger.

- You and your partner must agree to the procedure. Occasionally, infection can lead to failure. Failure in diabetic or immunosuppressed patients is more common. Mechanical problems with prostheses are rare.

- Penile prosthesis insertion requires a general or local anaesthetic. Antibiotics given during the operation will reduce the chance of infection. You will need to stay in hospital for 1–3 days and to take 1–2 weeks off work.

- The procedure is uncomfortable, taking 2–4 weeks to settle. You will be taught to pump an inflatable prosthesis at 4 weeks, which is when you will be able to have sexual intercourse. Other prostheses can also be used at 4 weeks.

24

Incisions for different penile prostheses

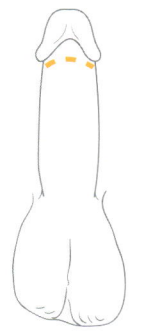

Subcoronal incision

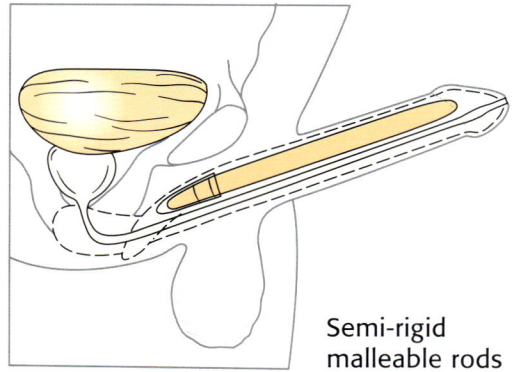

Semi-rigid
malleable rods

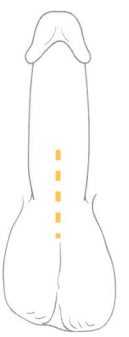

Penoscrotal incision

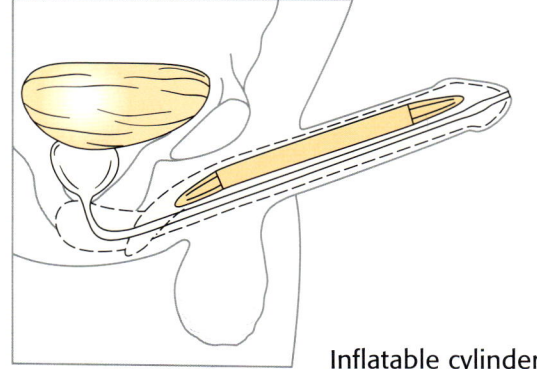

Inflatable cylinders

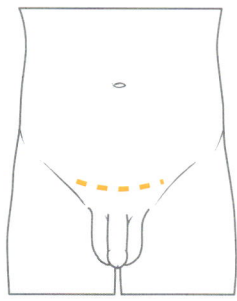

Infrapubic incision

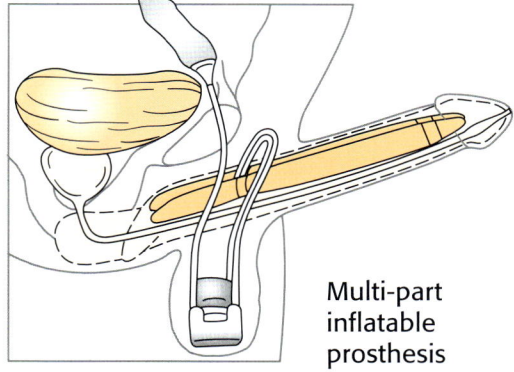

Multi-part
inflatable
prosthesis

Peyronie's disease: medical treatment and corporoplasty

- Peyronie's disease is a dense fibrous plaque in the erectile tissue that causes the penis to bend. Erections are usually still possible, but may be painful and can lead to erectile dysfunction.

- Peyronie's disease is usually a result of injury followed by tissue scarring. Your doctor will feel your penis to confirm Peyronie's disease. An intracavernosal injection of alprostadil is given to cause an erection, and a photograph taken to show the bend.

- Medical treatment is of limited value. Tamoxifen, an oral treatment, stops the initial inflammation and may relieve the early pain. Your urologist can inject drugs directly to soften and dissolve the plaque. A new therapy, extracorporeal shock wave therapy, appears to improve both pain and curvature.

- If your condition remains unchanged after 6 months, surgery is an option. In corporoplasty, also known as Nesbit's procedure, an erection is induced using a saline infusion. A tuck is made or a crescent-shaped piece of tissue removed opposite the plaque. The defect is then sewn transversely. Another erection is induced to check the correction has been made. This relatively minor procedure takes about 1 hour.

- You will need to stay in hospital overnight. Sexual intercourse is possible after 4 weeks and the procedure is successful in 80% of men. Some penile shortening occurs, but this is usually less than 2 cm. The bend may return and further surgery may be needed in the future.

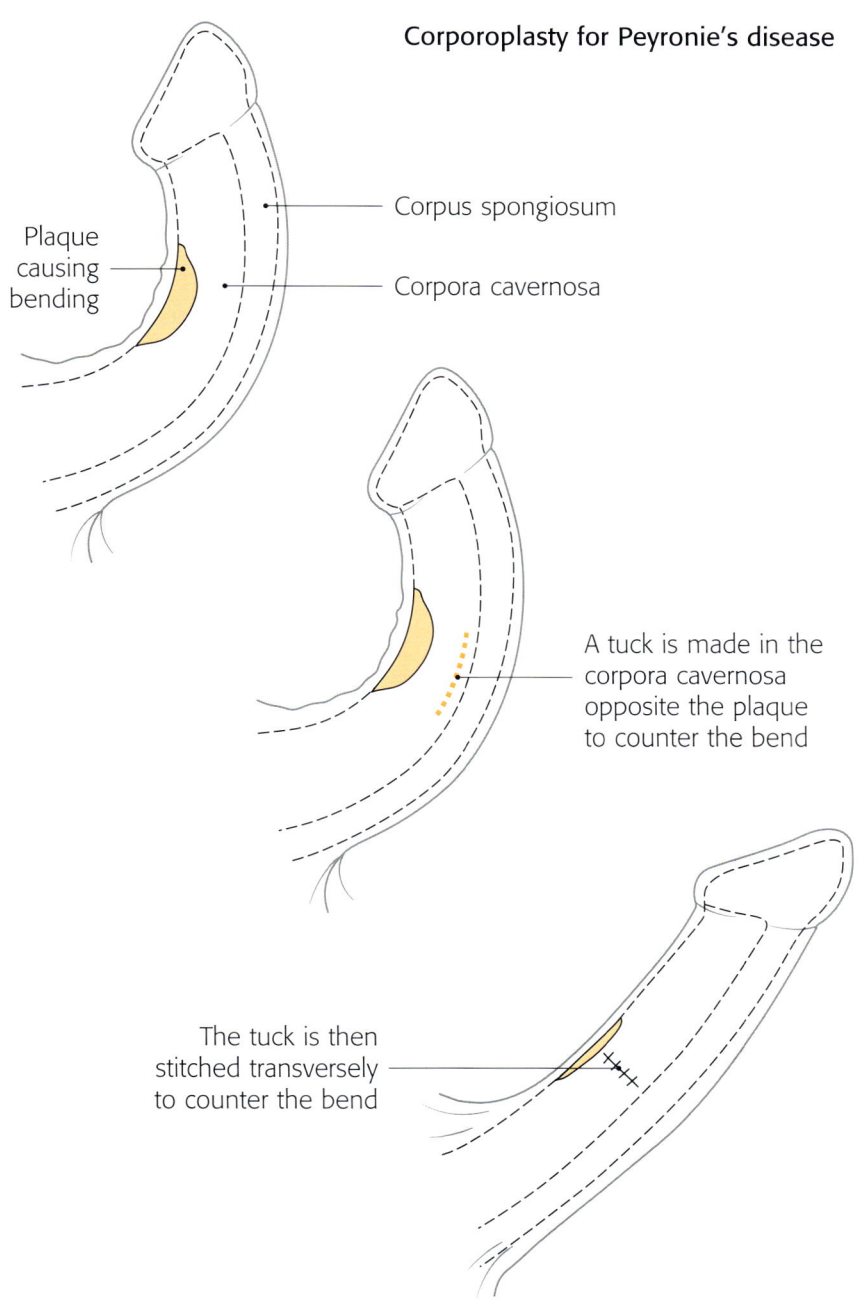

25

Corporoplasty for Peyronie's disease

Corpus spongiosum

Plaque causing bending

Corpora cavernosa

A tuck is made in the corpora cavernosa opposite the plaque to counter the bend

The tuck is then stitched transversely to counter the bend

Peyronie's disease: plaque incision and vein grafting

- If you have corporoplasty or Nesbit's procedure for Peyronie's disease and it is unsuccessful, you may need further surgery.

- Plaque incision and saphenous vein graft can be effective when corporoplasty has failed. This procedure does not cause further penile shortening. However, the neurovascular bundle can be damaged because it will need to be lifted off the plaque and you may lose sensation in the tip (glans) of the penis.

- It is possible for the plaque to be surgically removed. This is a more extensive procedure. The plaque is removed and the defect area can be filled with dermal graft, saphenous vein and synthetic material dacron. You will need to stay in hospital for 1 or 2 days, and can resume sexual intercourse after 4 weeks.

- If you have Peyronie's disease and a poor blood supply to the penis, a prosthesis can help. If an inflatable prosthesis is used, the plaque will need to be broken and reinforced cylinders inserted. You will need to stay in hospital for 1–3 days and can return to work after 1–2 weeks. After 4 weeks, you will be able to attempt sexual intercourse. Penile implants are very successful in this circumstance.

26

Plaque incision and vein grafting of Peyronie's disease

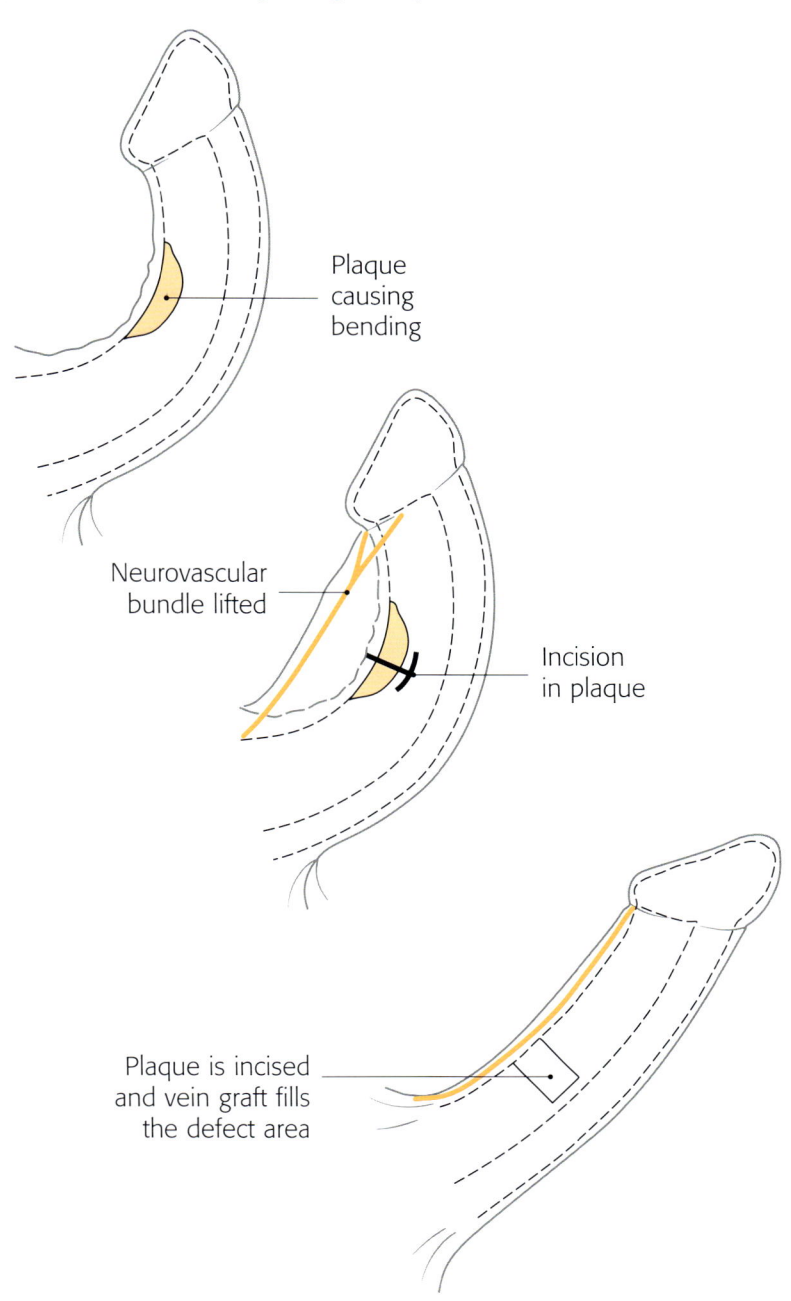

Plaque causing bending

Neurovascular bundle lifted

Incision in plaque

Plaque is incised and vein graft fills the defect area

Vascular surgery

- If your erectile dysfunction (ED) is due to a poor blood flow to the penis, vascular surgery can improve the blood flow or prevent blood leaking from the veins.

- Vascular surgery probably has only a limited role in the treatment of ED, and is often unsuccessful. Generally, it is most successful in young men who have had a pelvic fracture.

- Venous leakage is not likely to be a defect of the veins themselves. It may be due to the smooth muscle of the penis being unable to relax so that the penis does not fill with blood adequately. The operation for venous leakage – ligation and resection of the dorsal vein – has had very poor results and is now rarely performed. However, it is a relatively easy procedure and, unlike a penile prosthesis, means that you can benefit from future developments in treatment.

- The aim of the surgery is to improve the blood supply to the penis. An artery in the abdomen is redirected to the dorsal artery of the penis to increase the blood flow.

- However, you may require a penile prosthesis eventually.

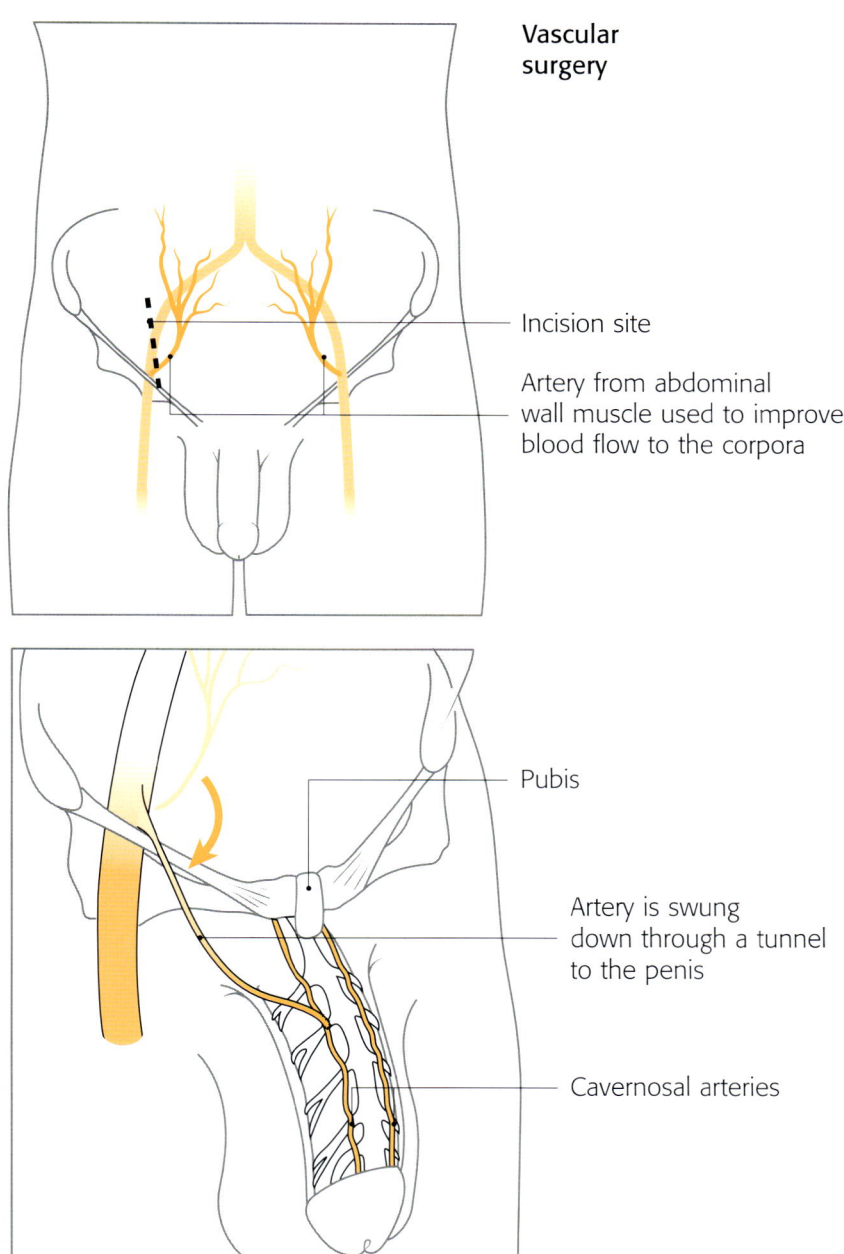

27

Vascular surgery

Incision site

Artery from abdominal wall muscle used to improve blood flow to the corpora

Pubis

Artery is swung down through a tunnel to the penis

Cavernosal arteries

Ejaculation disorders

- Approximately 10% of men attending sexual dysfunction clinics have problems with ejaculation rather than difficulty having erections.

- During ejaculation, the bladder neck closes and semen is expelled from the penis through the urethra. Semen consists of sperm produced in the testicles and fluid from the seminal vesicle and prostate gland.

- Retrograde ejaculation occurs when the bladder neck fails to close and semen passes into the bladder rather than coming out of the penis. Conditions that cause retrograde ejaculation include spina bifida, diabetes, neurological diseases and spinal injury. Up to 90% of men have retrograde ejaculation following surgery for prostate problems.

- Some drugs also cause retrograde ejaculation. These include alpha-blockers, which may be taken to treat symptoms of prostate enlargement, some drugs for high blood pressure and some antidepressants. Ejaculation usually returns to normal when you stop taking these drugs. However, never stop taking prescription drugs without first consulting your doctor.

- Sometimes it might be possible to overcome retrograde ejaculation by having intercourse with a full bladder.

- Retrograde ejaculation will not affect your health in any other way. Your semen will leave your bladder when you next pass urine.

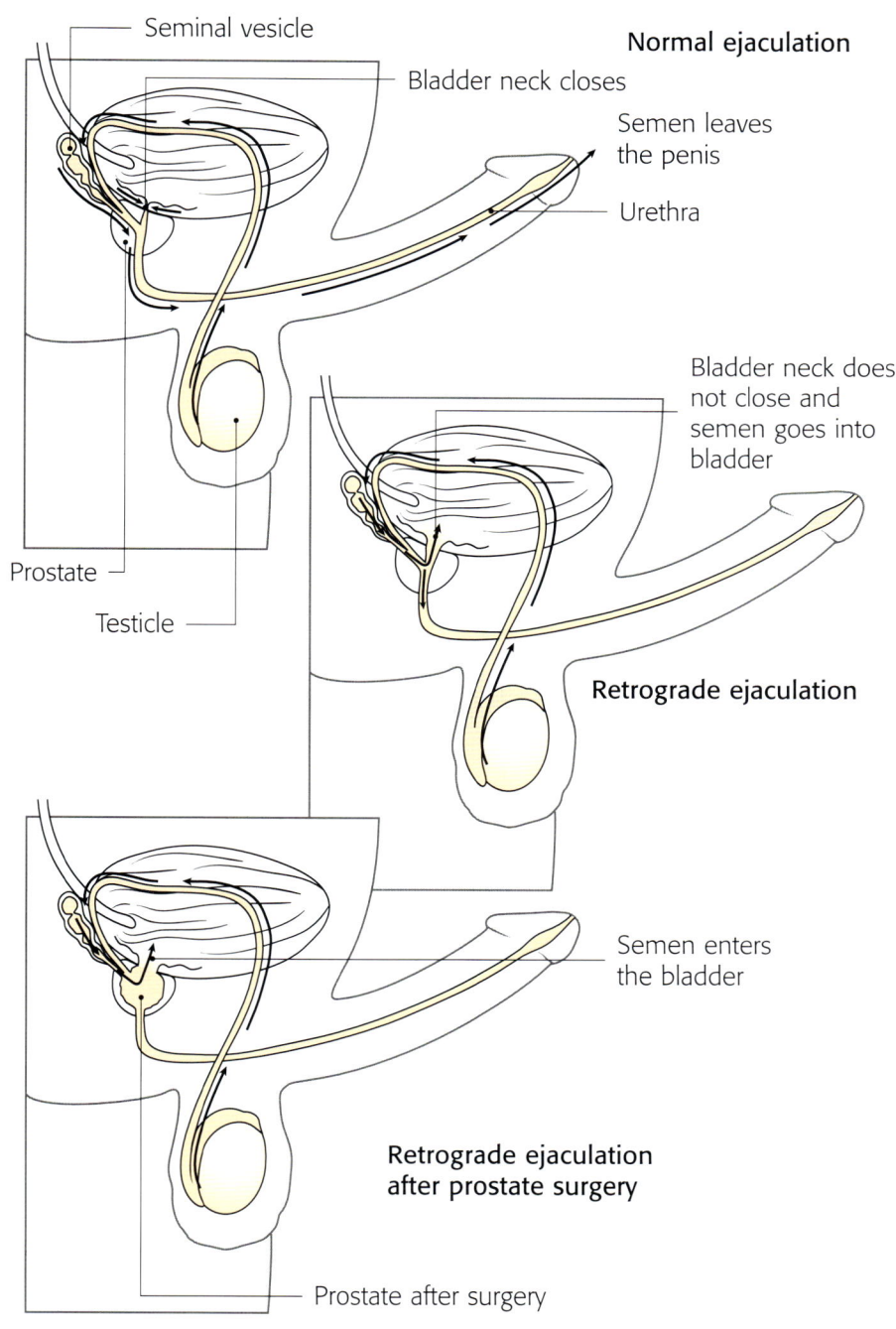

28

Seminal vesicle

Normal ejaculation

Bladder neck closes

Semen leaves
the penis

Urethra

Prostate

Testicle

Bladder neck does
not close and
semen goes into
bladder

Retrograde ejaculation

Semen enters
the bladder

**Retrograde ejaculation
after prostate surgery**

Prostate after surgery

Premature ejaculation

- If you reach orgasm before satisfying the needs of you or your partner, this is called premature ejaculation. Usually, it is due to psychological rather than physical causes. Other common sexual dysfunction problems associated with premature ejaculation include erectile dysfunction (ED) and loss of sex drive. By identifying and addressing the cause of your premature ejaculation, your ED is likely to improve.

- Premature ejaculation may be due to sexual problems in your female partner. If she has vaginismus (muscles around the vagina tighten suddenly), you are more likely to have ED and premature ejaculation. Vaginismus is treatable, so your partner should see her doctor.

- You can learn to recognize the stage in the orgasm cycle prior to ejaculation, but before it is inevitable, and prevent ejaculation by using the squeeze technique. When you feel as if you are about to ejaculate, you or your partner should compress the penis, where the shaft meets the glans, firmly but gently between the thumb and index finger. This pressure should be applied for 10–20 seconds. After letting go, do not do anything for about 30 seconds. Do this several times before allowing ejaculation to occur.

- Some types of antidepressant, in particular clomipramine and paroxetine, and local anaesthetic creams have been used successfully to treat premature ejaculation. These are taken or applied prior to sexual intercourse.

29

The squeeze technique for premature ejaculation

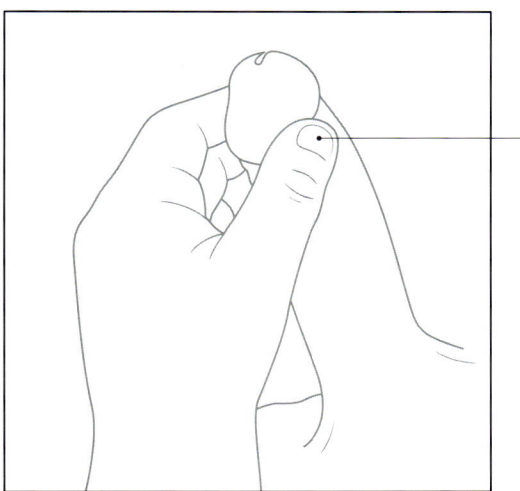

By applying pressure to the tip of the penis just before ejaculation, orgasm can be delayed

Anaesthetic cream, applied to the tip of the penis, can prevent premature ejaculation

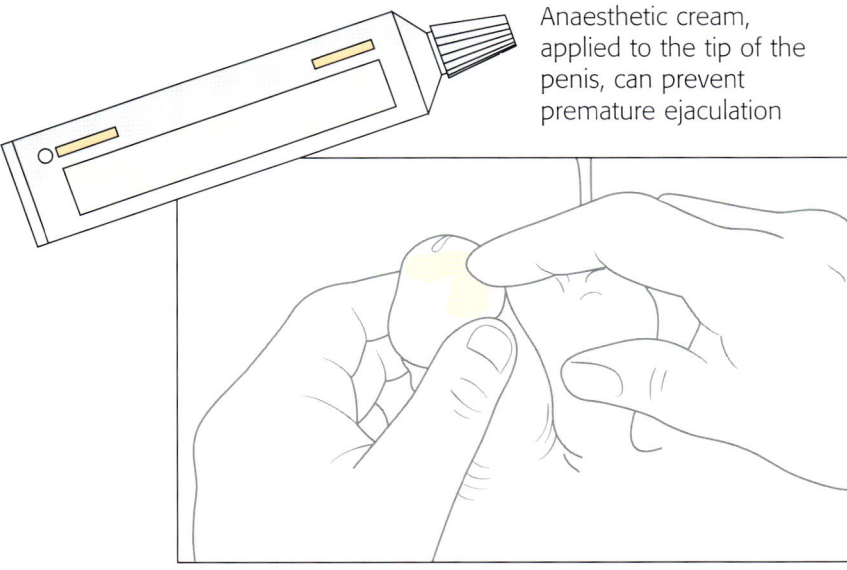

Anejaculation and painful ejaculation

- Some men achieve a successful erection, but do not ejaculate (anejaculation or anorgasmia). This may be due to problems with semen production or storage, or expulsion of semen down the urethra.

- An anatomical defect, such as an ejaculatory duct abnormality, may be the cause. More often, anejaculation follows pelvic surgery, spinal trauma or disease, or is due to an ejaculatory duct obstruction.

- Many prescription drugs can delay or prevent ejaculation. Drugs include those to treat high blood pressure, such as methyldopa, and antidepressants, such as paroxetine and amitriptyline. Your orgasm and ejaculation will usually return to normal when you stop taking the drug. Alcohol can also have a similar effect.

- Yohimbine, a plant extract, may be prescribed to treat anejaculation.

- Secondary, or acquired, anejaculation is more common, and is often a psychological problem. Your doctor can help you identify and address the causes.

- If you experience pain on ejaculation, you may have inflammation of the urethra, seminal vesicles or prostate.

- Investigations to check for sexually transmitted infections and other causes of urinary tract infections will be carried out. Urethral swabs will be taken and prostatic massage via the back passage (rectum) performed to look for any signs of infection.

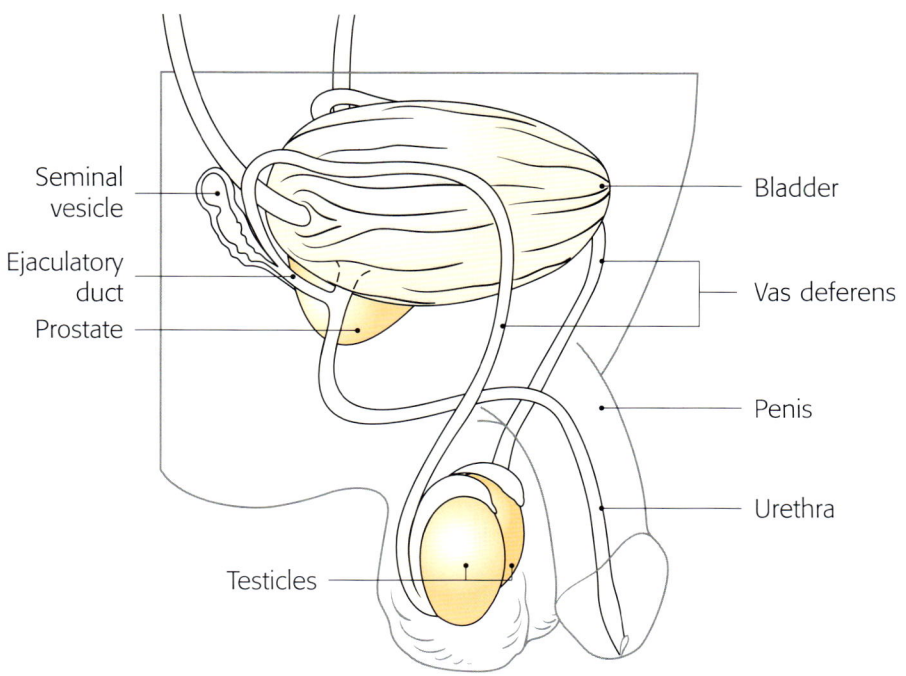

30

Seminal vesicle
Ejaculatory duct
Prostate
Bladder
Vas deferens
Penis
Urethra
Testicles

Reasons for anejaculation

- Ejaculatory duct abnormalities
- Psychological problems
- Inflammation of the urethra, prostate or seminal vesicles
- Drugs prescribed to treat other conditions

Priapism

- Priapism is a painful, prolonged erection, lasting more than 4 hours, in the absence of sexual desire. It can be caused by intracavernosal therapy, drugs such as trazodone, chlorpromazine or prazosin, conditions such as sickle-cell anaemia, leukaemia and metastatic cancer, and trauma.

- If left untreated, priapism can lead to permanently damaged erectile tissue. Priapism is a urological emergency and you must not delay seeking treatment.

- There are two types of priapism; low flow, the more common type, and high flow, which is very rare and is related to injury of the perineum (the area between the anus and the penis). High-flow priapism can occur intermittently.

- In low-flow priapism, the erection must be relieved within 12 hours. Under local anaesthetic, blood will be taken from the penis with a syringe to lower the pressure and relieve the discomfort. The corpora cavernosa are then flushed with saline to remove any blood clots. If this does not work, a drug (phenylephrine) can be given to narrow the blood vessels and reduce the blood flow to the penis. This will be repeated if necessary.

- If unsuccessful, surgery may be required. Surgery has a high initial success rate if priapism is treated within 24 hours. Surgery after 24 hours is likely to fail. The priapism can eventually lead to fibrosis, making recovery unlikely.

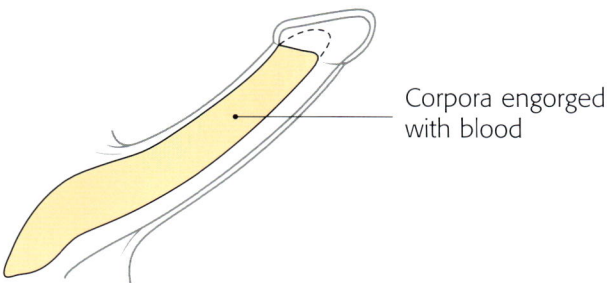

31

Priapism

Corpora engorged
with blood

Low-flow priapism

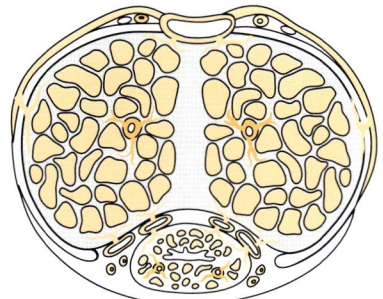

Large amounts of blood compress
the veins so blood cannot flow out

High-flow priapism

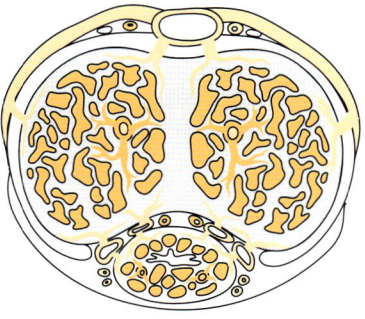

Large amounts of blood flow in
and out at a high rate

**Treating
priapism**

Blood
drawn off
and saline
flushed
through

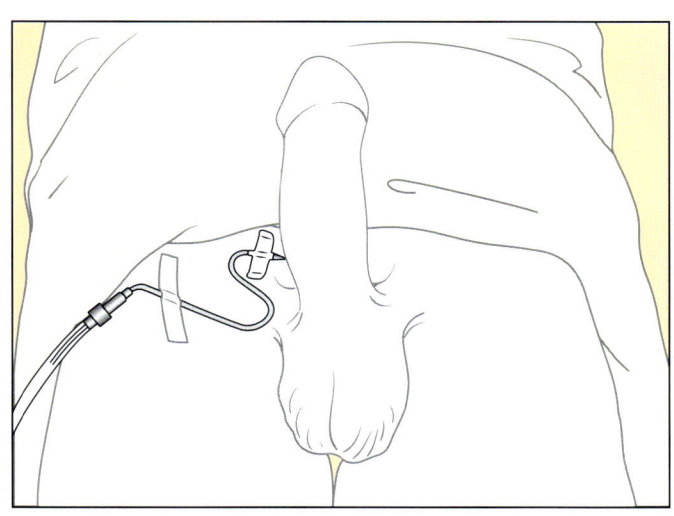

Penile lengthening

- An erect penis is 12–18 cm long; 13 cm is average. Penile lengthening is a treatment option if you have a webbed or buried penis, or an abnormally small penis (micropenis) that is less than 4 cm long when limp and less than 8–10 cm when erect.

- If you are distressed by the size of your penis, you should speak to your doctor. He will ask you questions about satisfactory relationships and sexual intercourse that you have had, and examine and measure your penis when limp and erect. Your doctor may suggest you speak to a psychosexual counsellor.

- The penile lengthening operation is performed under general anaesthetic. An incision is made above the pubis and the suspensory ligament, which holds the penis in place, is released. The operation takes about 1 hour, and you will need to take a month off work. You should be able to resume sexual intercourse after 4 weeks.

- After the operation, your erect penis will not move headwards and the base will be less secure. A weight may be applied to maintain the length. Repositioning fat around the spongy tissue in the penis can increase the girth. However, fat injections are not recommended as they can make the penis lumpy and deformed.

- Your penis will be a maximum of 2.5 cm longer. However, the appearance is not always good. The penis can retract and the neurovascular bundle may be damaged, making the glans numb.

32

Penile lengthening

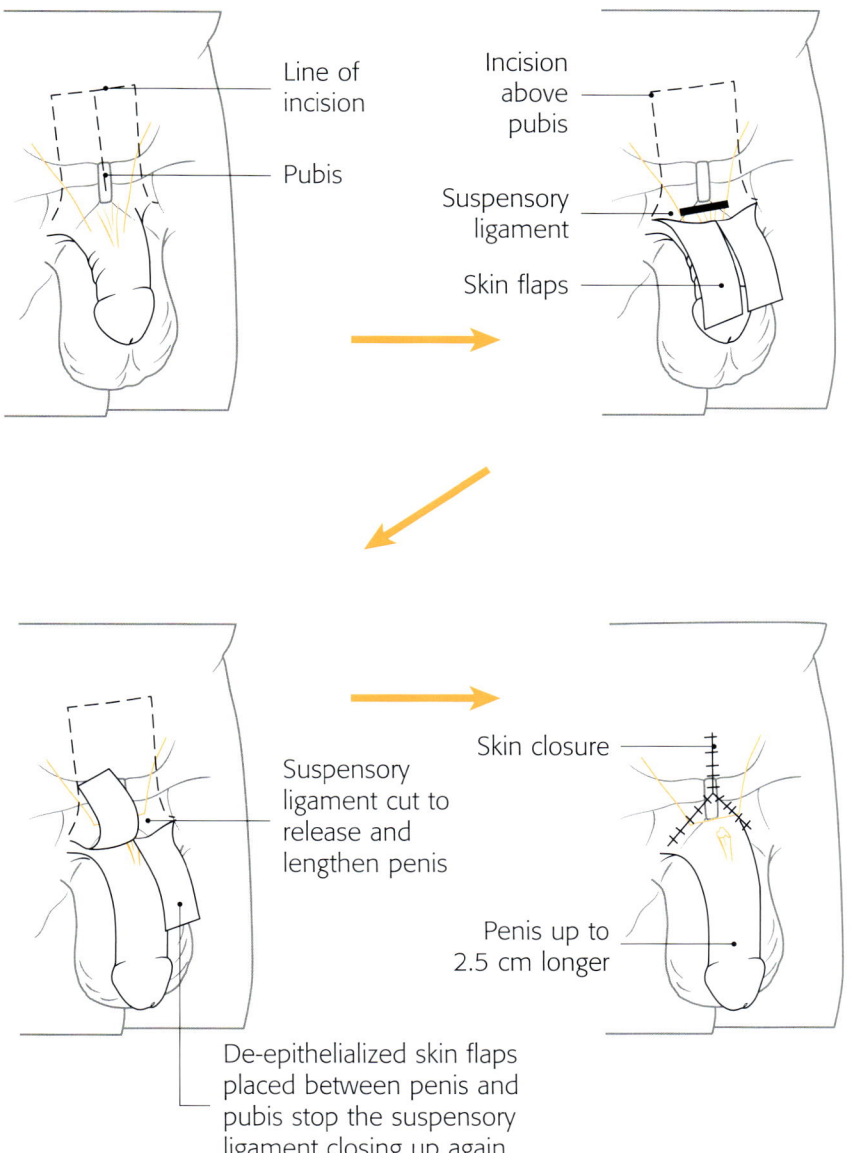

Line of incision

Pubis

Incision above pubis

Suspensory ligament

Skin flaps

Suspensory ligament cut to release and lengthen penis

Skin closure

Penis up to 2.5 cm longer

De-epithelialized skin flaps placed between penis and pubis stop the suspensory ligament closing up again